A Manual Of

Pravin Jaiprakash Gupta

A Manual Of Pilonidal Sinus Disease

Patient's plight, Doctor's dilemma

LAP LAMBERT Academic Publishing

Impressum / Imprint

Bibliografische Information der Deutschen Nationalbibliothek: Die Deutsche Nationalbibliothek verzeichnet diese Publikation in der Deutschen Nationalbibliografie; detaillierte bibliografische Daten sind im Internet über http://dnb.d-nb.de abrufbar.
Alle in diesem Buch genannten Marken und Produktnamen unterliegen warenzeichen-, marken- oder patentrechtlichem Schutz bzw. sind Warenzeichen oder eingetragene Warenzeichen der jeweiligen Inhaber. Die Wiedergabe von Marken, Produktnamen, Gebrauchsnamen, Handelsnamen, Warenbezeichnungen u.s.w. in diesem Werk berechtigt auch ohne besondere Kennzeichnung nicht zu der Annahme, dass solche Namen im Sinne der Warenzeichen- und Markenschutzgesetzgebung als frei zu betrachten wären und daher von jedermann benutzt werden dürften.

Bibliographic information published by the Deutsche Nationalbibliothek: The Deutsche Nationalbibliothek lists this publication in the Deutsche Nationalbibliografie; detailed bibliographic data are available in the Internet at http://dnb.d-nb.de.
Any brand names and product names mentioned in this book are subject to trademark, brand or patent protection and are trademarks or registered trademarks of their respective holders. The use of brand names, product names, common names, trade names, product descriptions etc. even without a particular marking in this works is in no way to be construed to mean that such names may be regarded as unrestricted in respect of trademark and brand protection legislation and could thus be used by anyone.

Coverbild / Cover image: www.ingimage.com

Verlag / Publisher:
LAP LAMBERT Academic Publishing
ist ein Imprint der / is a trademark of
AV Akademikerverlag GmbH & Co. KG
Heinrich-Böcking-Str. 6-8, 66121 Saarbrücken, Deutschland / Germany
Email: info@lap-publishing.com

Herstellung: siehe letzte Seite /
Printed at: see last page
ISBN: 978-3-659-29497-6

A MANUAL OF PILONIDAL SINUS DISEASE

PRAVIN JAIPRAKASH GUPTA,
MS, FICA, FICS, FASCRS, FAIS

Fine Morning Hospital and Research Center,
Laxmi Nagar, Nagpur- INDIA

CONTENTS

PREFACE   I-II

Chapter 1- INTRODUCTION TO PILONIDAL SINUS DISEASE   1

Chapter 2- PATHOPHYSIOLOGY OF PILONIDAL SINUS DISEASE

                                                            9

Chapter 3- PRESENTATIONS OF PILONIDAL SINUS DISEASE

                                                           18

Chapter 4- MANAGEMENT OF PILONIDAL SINUS DISEASE

                                                           28

Chapter 5- SURGICAL TREATMENT OF PILONIDAL SINUS
           DISEASE

                                                           44

Chapter 6- OTHER PILONIDAL SINUS DISEASES

                                                           87

ACKNOWLEDGEMENT   101

PREFACE

Like all other branches of learning, medicine and surgery has been, and is, a living organism having self-propelling powers of expansion and innovations. The search for cost effective, time effective and patient-friendly solutions for ameliorating the sufferings of the masses has always been a continuous pursuit of the medical practitioners.

Pilonidal Sinus Disease is one of the most important branches of medical practice because of its complexities and which often is mired by misguiding symptoms. This ailment is often found affecting young and healthy people.

As they say, every patient afflicted even with a known disease is a challenge for the physician and surgeon for no single treatment modality could be the answer for effectively treating his very typical symptoms and his constitution. It is here that the expertise of the surgeon based on his experience is on test. He has to choose from among numerous non-surgical and surgical procedures in vogue suitable to the exacting requirement of the particular patient. The aim, obviously, is to provide maximum relief to and to ensure most patient satisfaction while meticulously avoiding the chances of treatment failure, recurrence and morbidity. The surgeon has also to take care of the economics of the treatment, minimum hospital stay and early return to work, more so in the developing and under-developed countries. This is where the surgeon is supposed to set the gold standard by carefully choosing a patient-specific single or a combination of treatment procedures available to him.

In this book I have attempted to discuss the pathogenesis of pilonidal sinus disease and a variety of treatment modalities available for acute pilonidal abscesses, small sinus tracts, and complex or recurrent pilonidal disease. The book also elaborates on the disease encountered at a few uncommon yet important sites.

I express my heartfelt gratefulness to the doyens of this noble profession who, over periods, have painstakingly invented and successfully practiced different surgical and non-surgical procedures in combating this nagging disease. I have made no attempt to provide a comprehensive bibliography. This is not a text book, but a manual of this complex disease.

31st October, 2012   Dr. Pravin J. Gupta

Chapter 1

INTRODUCTION TO PILONIDAL SINUS

DISEASE

Pilonidal disease is an infection under the skin in the gluteal cleft. It affects an estimated 26 per 100,000 persons, occurring primarily in young adults with a 3:1 male predilection. Known risk factors include family history, local trauma, sedentary occupation, and obesity.

Pilonidal sinus disease (PSD) consists of a symptom complex with presentation that ranges from asymptomatic pits to painful draining lesions that are predominantly located in sacrococcygeal region.

Though it is not life threatening, yet it remains troublesome, disabling nuisance and an embarrassing disease condition with considerable discomfort and morbidity.

At times, it may be seen at body locations other than the sacrococcygeal region and can rarely manifest with serious complications like infections or leading to fatality particularly when carcinogenic changes occur.

In 1833, Herbert Mayo described this entity for the first time. Mayo's findings were of a characteristic epithelial track (the sinus) that generally contained hair and was located in the skin of the natal cleft. In 1880, Hodge suggest the term "pilonidal" (Latin: *pilus* = hair and *nidus* = nest), to indicate a disease consisting of hair-containing sinus in the sacrococcygeal area. Buie noted its prevalence in male, military recruits who drove jeeps and thus characterized it as "jeep disease" (Fig.1). Pilonidal disease was most notable during World

War II when an estimated 80,000 soldiers became afflicted and lost significant time from active duty.

The soldiers observed a common association of the problem with driving military vehicles especially the Jeep. In the Jeep, the driver sat with the thighs flexed forcing his flattened sacral region into the canvas seat. The vehicle's suspension was basic. Travel over rough ground caused excessive friction and this was thought to force hairs into the skin.

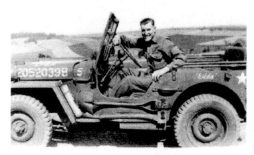

Figure 1- The Jeep Disease

PSD remains a common problem of sacrococcygeal region occurring in the cleavage between buttocks (natal cleft), and is often called as primary sacrococcygeal pilonidal disease: **SPD**. However, **PSD** is not restricted to inter-gluteal region alone but may occur in inter-digital space, hand, axilla, peri-umbilical areas, in the scalp, in the penile and subungual region. For many years, the cause of sacrococcygeal pilonidal sinus (**SPD**) has been a matter of debate, when it was thought to be congenital, but which is now being well recognized as an acquired condition as Patey & Scarf proposed in 1946 (Fig.2).

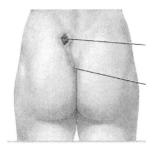

Figure 2- Pilonidal sinus tract and wound

In the nineteenth century, basing their theories on the study of the human embryo, many authors proposed a congenital origin of the lesion.

These theories suggested that this entity might be caused by:

1. Persistence of a caudal remnant of the neural canal that remained adherent to the cutaneous surface, forming small cysts which later rupture, causing blind-ended sinuses.

2. Dermal inclusions caused by cystic changes of sequestered epithelial rests.

3. Dermoid tractions created during involution of human tail bud - a lack of development of the caudal appendix attracts the skin into a subcutaneous area resulting in an epithelium-lined tract.

4. Preen gland-like structures considered to be a phylogenetic representation of the preen gland or "scent" gland found in the

sacrococcygeal region of some species of birds, which empty through a duct in the skin of the posterior region were thought to be special down growths of epithelium originating from the skin.

The opponents of the congenital origin of this condition state the following:

1. The presence of developmental abnormalities similar to those in sacrococcygeal region in the cervical and dorsal areas of the vertebral column unaccompanied by pilonidal sinus.

2. The presence of the entity in males more than females while in congenital aspects an equal ratio is expected.

3. Its appearance in the adolescence period of life is not in accordance with a developmental defect.

4. The linkage between pilonidal disease and occupation e.g. among Jeep-driver soldiers and on barbers' hands.

5. The description of similar lesions in other sites of the body.

6. The lack of hair follicles and other skin appendages in the wall of the sinuses despite the presence of hair shafts, freely and deeply embedded in granulation tissue or scar and the lack of lining epithelium in most cases were important histological factors that added criticism to the congenital theories.

In addition, there is a high recurrence rate of **PSD** after surgical excision. These factors argue against the validity of the congenital theory to explain **PSD**. Further, congenital tracts do not contain hair and are lined by cuboidal epithelium.

PSD are reported more frequently from the Western world (Caucasians) than from Asia and Africa and is also common in Turkey and Egypt. It is widely prevalent in western countries like

Denmark, Switzerland, Italy, Germany, UK and in USA. Current report showed that 40000 **PSD** patients are treated each year in civilian hospitals in USA which average 5.2 days of in-hospital care. **PSD** is also common in several countries of Arabian Peninsula and the gulf like Kuwait, Jordan and Saudi Arabia.

Pilonidal disease in the general population has a male preponderance. It occurs in the ratio of 3 or 4:1. In children, however, the ratio is the opposite occurring in 4 females for each male it afflicts. Pilonidal disease commonly affects adults in the second to third decade of life. Pilonidal sinus diseases are extremely uncommon after age 40 years, and the incidence usually decreases by age 25 years. The average age of presentation is 21 years for men and 19 years for women.

Males are affected more frequently probably due to their more hirsute nature. Proportionately, females make up a quarter of those undergoing hospital treatments, possibly reflecting under-reporting in the male population. The condition is more common in whites than Asians or Africans due to differing hair characteristics and growth patterns. In a study of risk factors the following associations were found;

- sedentary occupation -44%
- positive family history - 38%
- obesity - 50%
- local irritation or trauma prior to onset of symptoms - 34%.

Few other factors implicated in its etiology are large buttocks with deep natal cleft, folliculitis at another site, occupations requiring prolonged sitting, traveling or driving, excessive body hair, and poor local hygiene. The fact that so many men doing the same sort of job developed pilonidal sinuses suggests that environmental factors might be playing an important role in the development of the condition. Examples of such factors included wearing restrictive clothing, such as army uniforms and repetitive motion, such as bouncing around on the seat of a jeep or back of the camel.

Hair is the main initiative agent in all theories that attempt to explain the pathogenesis of **PSD**, which may be the reason for the male predomination of the disease. Hair is the invader agent. Clinical observations also revealed that patients with **PSD** are usually hairy men. Increasing body hair rate was matched to 9.23-fold higher risk of **PSD** even after adjustment for other risk factors. The incidence of pilonidal disease is also affected by hair characteristics, such as kinking, medullation, coarseness, and growth rate.

In one study evaluating the relation between the bathing habituation and **PSD**, it was hypothesized that this relation affected the amount of loose hair at the intergluteal groove. The adjusted risk of **PSD** diagnosis is 6.33-fold greater for those who bath two or less times per week than the risk for those people who take three or more baths per week. The results revealed that regular cleaning of intergluteal sulcus may prevent this disease.

Current makes of cars and trucks are comfortable and roads are flat. It is possible that improved vehicle and road conditions are the reason today's drivers experience **PSD** less often than with their colleagues who rode in a jumping jeep on bumpy field roads during the Second World War. Nonetheless, occupation seems to be indirectly related to sitting time and body cleaning.

Sitting time in a day on a seat is another risk factor evaluated. The adjusted risk of **PSD** is 4.3-fold higher for individuals who were sitting more than six hours in a day. The majority of the classical articles about **PSD** indicate a relation between the long sitting time and this disease.

Recent studies have found that obesity is a relatively less important risk factor for **PSD**. The intergluteal groove is a deep moist area in which broken hairs and foreign bodies can collect, leading to infection or invasion of the skin. The deepness of the intergluteal sulcus may be different in people based on BMI or personal body characteristics.

Points to Ponder-

PSD can present either as a chronic discharging sinus tract or as an acute abscess. The etiology of **PSD** remains controversial, and, although long held to be a congenital condition, emerging evidence is in favor of it being an acquired condition. Obstruction of the hair follicles leads to their enlargement and eventual rupture, leading to abscess and sinus formation. This may be perpetuated by the entry of loose hairs into the skin pits. Male gender, obesity, occupations or sports requiring sitting, a deep natal cleft, excessive body hair, stiff or coarse hair, poor body hygiene and excessive sweating are described as the primary risk factors for **PSD**.

Further reading and references

1.   Mayo OH. Observations on Injuries and Diseases of the Rectum. London: Burgess and Hill; 1833.

2.   Hodges RM. Pilonidal sinus. Boston Med Surg J 1880; 103: 485–486.

3.   Buie LA. Jeep disease. South Med J 1944; 37:103–109.

4.   Gage M. Pilonidal sinus: an explanation of its embryologic development. Arch Surg. 1935; 31:175-89.

5.   Patey DH, Scarff RW. Pathology of postanal pilonidal sinus: it's bearing on treatment. Lancet. 1946; 2:484-6.

6.   Brearley R. Pilonidal sinus. A new theory of origin. Br J Surg. 1955; 43:455-62.

7.   Classic articles in colonic and rectal surgery. Louis A. Buie, M.D. 1890-1975: Jeep disease (pilonidal disease of mechanized warfare). Dis Colon Rectum. 1982; 25:384-90.

8.   Franckowiak JJ, Jackman RJ. The etiology of pilonidal sinus. Dis Colon Rectum 1962;5:28–36

9.   Hardaway RM. Pilonidal cyst—neither pilonidal nor cyst. Arch Surg 1958; 76:143–147.

10.   Søndenaa K, Andersen E, Nesvik I, Søreide JA. Patient characteristics and symptoms in chronic pilonidal sinus disease. Int J Colorectal Dis 1995; 10:39– 42.

Chapter 2

PATHOPHYSIOLOGY OF PILONIDAL SINUS DISEASE

Pilonidal sinus disease presents either as a draining sinus or as an abscess. There is an underlying cyst like-structure with associated granulation tissue, fibrosis & frequent tufts of hair. Moreover, this sinus is initiated from a small midline opening lined by stratified squamous epithelium. Hair maintains an adverse environment within the natal cleft aggravating PSD and that pits presenting into dermis are distended with keratin & debris.

Bascom examined midline pits in the natal cleft microscopically and concluded that they are enlarged and distorted hair follicles. The cause of formation of these distorted hair follicles is unclear. Gravity and motion of the gluteal folds have been suggested as a cause of creation of a vacuum that pulls on the follicles (Fig.1).

Local inflammation by bacteria, debris and edema, which occludes the mouth of the follicle, leads to further expansion of the follicle which then ruptures resulting in a foreign body reaction and micro abscesses which then develop into acute and chronic pilonidal abscesses along with laterally displaced and epithelized tracts. Once the micro abscess becomes a burrowing infection, the disease is defined as a pilonidal sinus.

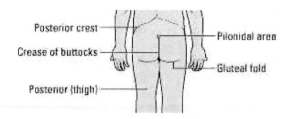

Figure 1- Anatomical description of the pilonidal area

Acquired pilonidal sinus often results from an in-growing hair, which leads to the hair follicle becoming distended with keratin and infected due to the accumulation of hair, cellular debris and bacteria. Once a hair follicle starts to become blocked, an inflammatory reaction follows where localized edema causes the pore to close. This can be assisted by natural movement of the skin. The built up of purulent material eventually creates pressure, which leads to leakage into the surrounding tissues. The hair itself becomes a foreign body, which accentuates the inflammatory response (Fig.2).

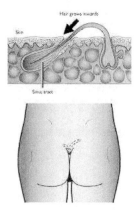

Figure 2- Hair invasion process in the pilonidal sinus

The etiology of pilonidal disease as a foreign body reaction is supported by histological examination. It demonstrates foreign body giant cells associated with hair shafts that are embedded in chronic granulation tissue lining the abscess cavity and sinus tracts.

Although only 50%–75% of cysts or sinuses contain hair shafts during exploration, hair has three important distinct roles. First, de novo hair in the distended hair follicle can remain unshed and enhance micro abscess formation. Second, free hairs from other parts of the body can invade the follicle's open mouth and creating foreign body reaction. Third, skin hair in close vicinity to pilonidal wound irritates it mechanically, affecting healing.

In dealing with the pathogenesis of pilonidal sinus disease, Karydakis attributed the hair insertion process to three main factors:

1. The invader, which is the loose hair,

2. The force, which causes the insertion, and

3. The vulnerability of the skin to the insertion of hair at the depth of the natal cleft.

He also identified secondary factors and expressed these in an equation. Some of these factors had been postulated earlier, but Karydakis showed their relevance in formulating a successful surgical approach. These two theories by Bascom and Karydakis offer the best explanations of pathogenesis of pilonidal sinus disease.

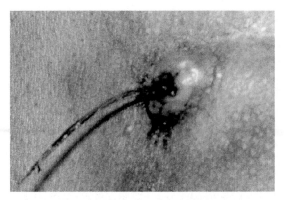

Figure 3- Extruding hairs from the sinus

Pathology

The sinus is initiated from a small midline opening lined by stratified squamous epithelium. Additional sinuses are frequent and have lateral openings. Cyst cavities may contain hair shafts, epithelial debris, and young granulation tissue. The sinus is lined by granulation tissue, infiltrated by neutrophils, lymphocytes, plasma cells, and sometimes hemosiderin laden macrophages.

Foreign body giant cells in association with dead hairs are also a frequent finding. Hair shafts are seen in 50%–75% of pilonidal sinuses lying free in the cavity or embedded in granulation tissue or deeply in a scar tissue (Fig.3). Occasionally, there is no visible opening or only a depression. Cutaneous appendages (hair follicles, sweat or sebaceous glands, and musculi arrectores pilorum) are not usually found in the wall of sinuses. Malignant transformation is rare but cases of squamous cell carcinoma and verrucous carcinoma have been reported.

Pilonidal disease starts at the onset of puberty, when sex hormones start acting on pilosebaceous glands in the natal cleft. A hair follicle becomes distended with keratin- and subsequently infected, leading to a folliculitis and an abscess down into the subcutaneous fat. Tracts spread out of the cavity in the directions of the neighboring hair growths, which in 90% of cases is towards the patient's head. Small proportions have tracts which pass caudally, and these pilonidal sinuses tend to be closer to the anus. Hairs are drilled or sucked into the cavity owning to friction with movements of the buttocks. Barbs on the hair prevent their expulsion, so they become trapped provoking a foreign body type reaction and infection (Fig.4).

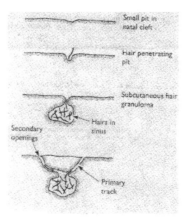

Figure 4- Formation of tract and secondary openings in the sinus cavity

The built up of purulent material eventually creates pressure, leading to creep into the surrounding tissues. The hair itself acts a foreign body, which accentuates the inflammatory response. The resultant micro-abscesses can become infected with bacteria, which release toxins that destroy tissue in the wound. The affected area becomes flooded with neutrophils and macrophages as the body's inflammatory response begins. This can result in the area becoming edematous and this will present as a cellulitis, which can be very painful. The built up of purulent material can result in its drainage onto the surface of the skin (Fig.5).

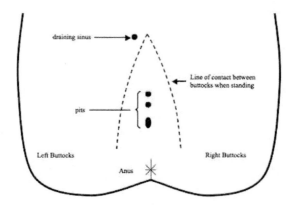

Figure 5- Progression of the infective process

Eventually, the follicle and the inflamed tissues can become a chronic abscess, prone to recurrent infection due to the combination of moisture, bacteria, hair and friction. In rare cases, due to the constant damage and repair cycle, malignancy can result and, although uncommon, it should be considered a potential complication in this patient group.

Follicular hyperplasia/hyperkeratosis and interfollicular epidermal hyperplasia are main features of PSD. Early pathology seems to take place at terminal hair follicles, whereas sinus tract formations are a secondary event. Focused regions show an inflammatory mixed infiltrate consisting of CD3+, CD4+, CD8+, CD68+ and CD79+ cells.

Bacteriology

Various studies have confirmed the polymicrobial nature and predominance of anaerobic bacteria in infected pilonidal sinuses, where they outnumbered aerobes. Gram negative aerobic and facultative bacilli, especially E coli, Proteus, and Pseudomonas are isolated in many instances. Staphylococci are only occasionally recovered.

The recovery of Gram negative bacilli is common. The predominant anaerobic isolates are Bacteroides, anaerobic cocci, Clostridium, and Fusobacterium. The predominant aerobes include E coli and group D streptococcus. Various Bacteroides, including B fragilis, anaerobic Gram positive cocci, and Clostridium have also been isolated.

The synergy among the different bacterial strains in mixed polymicrobial aerobic and anaerobic infections may be due to protection from phagocytosis and intracellular killing, production of essential growth factors, and lowering of oxidation reduction potential in infected host tissues.

The isolation of anaerobic bacteria mixed with aerobic and facultative organisms at that site is not surprising as anaerobes are the predominant organisms in the gastrointestinal tract, where they outnumber aerobes by 1000:1. Because anaerobic bacteria are often associated with pilonidal sinuses, physicians should consider their presence while using antibiotics. Gram staining of aspirated pus and appropriate aerobic and anaerobic microbiological techniques can help in the selection of proper treatment.

As some of the anaerobes are resistant to penicillin, treatment should also include appropriate coverage of those organisms. The presence of penicillin resistant anaerobic bacteria, however, such as B fragilis and some strains of the B melaninogenicus group may warrant the administration of appropriate antimicrobial agents such as clindamycin, cefoxitin, metronidazole, imipenem, or the combination of a B lactamase inhibitor and penicillin.

Points to Ponder-

Although often described incorrectly as a cyst, pilonidal cavities are not true cysts and lack a fully epithelized lining; but at times, the fibrous tracts of the sinus may be epithelized. Pilonidal sinus or disease is therefore the correct term. The majority of sinus tracts extend cephalad; but, additional sinuses may branch laterally.

Hair follicles may or may not be seen on pathologic examination. Cavities may contain hair, debris, and granulation tissue. The local cellular infiltration is sizable and often includes foreign body giant cells in association with hair.

Further reading and references

1.   Bascom J. Pilonidal sinus: origin from follicles of hairs and results of follicle removal as treatment. Surgery. 1980; 87:567-72.

2.   Karydakis GE. New approach to the problem of pilonidal sinus. Lancet. 1973; 2(7843):1414–1415.

3.   Doll D, Friederichs J, Dettmann H, Boulesteix AL, Duesel W, Petersen S. Time and rate of sinus formation in pilonidal sinus disease. Int J Colorectal Dis. 2008; 23:359-64.

4.   da Silva JH. Pilonidal cyst: cause and treatment. Dis Colon Rectum. 2000; 43:1146-56.

5.   Cubukçu A, Carkman S, Gönüllü NN, Alponat A, Kayabaşi B, Eyüboğu E. Lack of evidence that obesity is a cause of pilonidal sinus disease. Eur J Surg. 2001; 167:297-8.

6.   Classic articles in colonic and rectal surgery. Louis A. Buie, M.D. 1890-1975: Jeep disease (pilonidal disease of mechanized warfare). Dis Colon Rectum. 1982; 25:384-90.

7.   Jones D. Pilonidal sinus. BMJ 1992; 305:410–412.

8.   Mallory FB. Sacro-coccygeal dimples, sinuses and cysts. Am J Med Sci 1892; 103: 263–277.

9.   Marrie TJ, Aylwarad D, Kerr E, et al. Bacteriology of pilonidal cyst abscesses. J Clin Pathol 1978; 31:909.

10.   Brook I. Aerobic and anaerobic microbiology of pilonidal cyst abscesses in children. Am J Dis Child 1980; 134:679-80.

Chapter 3

PRESENTATION OF PILONIDAL DISEASE

A pilonidal sinus may present in a number of ways, ranging from acute illness with high levels of pain to a painful area in the coccyx region. It can present acutely as a pilonidal abscess, asymptomatically as a small pit or non-tender lump, or as a discharging lesion with or without pain or a lump. Examination reveals the characteristic opening in the natal cleft, through which a tuft of hair may be popping out at times. Affected person tend to be younger, which is consistent with their earlier onset of puberty. Patients are usually, but not invariably, dark and hairy, and are often obese.

Clinical presentations of pilonidal sinus can have four disease 'stages':

1. Asymptomatic — an initial stage pilonidal sinus may be discovered by the patient himself or on routine medical examination.

2. Acute — this will present as a painful, swollen area with a sacrococcygeal abscess, which may have purulent exudates. There may also be cellulitis over the natal cleft (Fig.1). Half of all patients present with an abscess and can present with progressive discomfort or pain after physical activity or a period of prolonged sitting, such as during a long drive or with obvious acute purulent drainage, pain, and swelling. Spontaneous drainage often occurs, to be followed by

generally painless chronic waxing and waning drainage from the secondary sinuses. Most patients present initially with pain, tenderness, swelling, and erythema in the gluteal cleft with or without drainage from the involved area. Primary pits may be visible in the midline of the gluteal cleft; however, they are often obscured. If observed, the diagnosis of pilonidal disease is supported. Symptoms related to pilonidal abscess include fever, chills, and pain, and intermittent discharge or bleeding is common from sinus tracts. Affected patients are typically in their middle to late 20's and have had symptoms for 4 to 5 years at initial presentation.

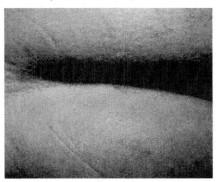

Figure 1- Cellulitis in the sacrococcygeal region

3.   Chronic — this will manifest as recurrent infections in the sacrococcygeal area. The patient complains of recurrent episodes of pain or sepsis. There are often periods of several months between episodes. As the size of the sinus increases the frequency of painful episodes also increases.

4.   Infected post-operative wound.

Pilonidal disease is a clinical diagnosis. Location is the easiest way to distinguish pilonidal disease from other disease entities.

Majority of patients present with an acute abscess cephalad in the natal cleft. This position distinguishes the disease from other common anorectal problems such as perirectal abscesses and anal fistulae, which are typically found near the anus. Midline pits are the distinguishing feature, occurring in 100% of cases, and these can typically be identified 4 to 8 cm from the anus. The application of pressure on the surrounding skin may lead to emission of pus from the openings. The secondary orifices are more or less lateral to the intergluteal sulcus. During the stage of inactivity, these orifices may be so tiny so as to be overlooked on primary inspection.

One may find some pits in the sulcus between the buttocks which may communicate with the sinus. By palpation it is possible to find an irregular induration between the primary and secondary orifices.

Hair within the abscess cavity is present in approximately two thirds of cases in men and one third of those in woman. As the acute abscess resolves, whether spontaneously or with treatment, chronic sinus tracts develop toward the skin. Chronic or recurrent abscesses with extensive branching sinus tracts develop in a small minority of patients. This complex variant of the disease may stem from prolonged neglect of symptoms but also occurs despite appropriate treatment.

Patients with PSD may complain about tiny pits or pores at the bottom of their back. Pain or discomfort during sit up is another worry. A tender or non tender zone may be present at the affected site. Only one fifth of the patients will present with acute pain and discomfort while four-fifth will have intermittently draining sinuses ranging between wetness to frank flow. Often the area will drain fluid that may be clear, cloudy or bloody. The openings could range from one to fifteen, or there may be a slit with pounding granulation ending in a cavity (Fig.2).

Hairs may be seen projecting from the openings and could be single or as a tuft and may be unduly long at times. Unhealed wound may be seen with a bridge of weak skin with underlying cavity filled with granulation tissue.

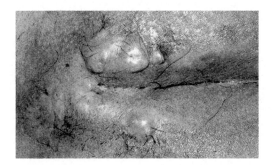

Figure 2- Lateral and midline sinuses

Occasionally, a history of trauma is recalled, and the patient may state that a similar lesion occurred in that area before, for which the patient may have had a primary incision and drainage or other definitive care prior to this presentation.

Given that most patients are young and healthy, other co-morbidities are not common, and review of systems is often negative, including fever and chills.

The physical findings in pilonidal disease are dependent on the stage of disease at presentation. In the early stages, the patient can notice a sinus tract or pit in the sacrococcygeal region. This can progress to midline edema or abscess formation (Fig.3). As with any abscess, physical examination findings include tenderness to palpation, fluctuance, warmth, purulent discharge, and induration or cellulitis.

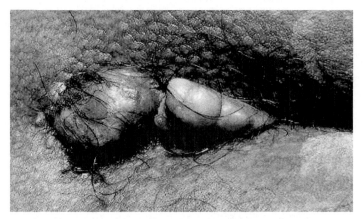

Figure 3- Recurrent pilonidal sinuses with abscess

The diagnostic examination must be completed by a digital and anoscopic examination to exclude suppurative anal lesions. The openings may be probed to know the direction of the sinus. Diagnosis is usually clear on history and examination alone though there may be some doubt in cases in which direction of the sinus is caudal creating a confusion of being a fistula in ano.

Differential Diagnosis of Pilonidal sinus disease

The differential diagnosis of pilonidal disease includes anorectal cryptoglandular abscess extending into the natal cleft, hidradenitis, and low anorectal fistula such as seen in Crohn's disease. A digital rectal examination with a rigid proctoscopy should therefore be performed prior to operating upon a patient for pilonidal disease.

In acute stage, an ischiorectal abscess may be mistaken for a pilonidal, but the former usually presents a definite systemic reaction. The origin of an ischiorectal abscess is almost always within the anorectal canal, and the abscess itself is merely a stage in the development of an anorectal fistula. From its position and tenderness in the anal or rectal canal, and the discovery of an internal opening at or near the anorectal line, the diagnosis is clear.

A fistula-in-ano is shown by probing, proctoscopy and sigmoidoscopy. It should be noted that the mid-line pilonidal sinus always goes deep and cranially. Boils, carbuncles, infected sebaceous cysts, neither give the characteristic prolonged history, nor that of repeated attacks. Other conditions to keep in mind are osteomyelitis and tuberculosis of the sacrum, which can be ruled out by X-ray examination.

Actinomycosis may occur in this area and is to be excluded by bacteriological examination. Inclusion dermoids, chordomas, teratomas and other neoplasms also need to be considered. In the great majority of cases of pilonidal sinus, careful search will reveal one or more characteristic mid-line openings, and if hair, as in the occasional cases, is seen protruding from the sinus it will make the diagnosis obvious.

Pyoderma gangrenosum and hidradenitis suppurativa are the two prominent conditions which may contain hair shafts.

Usually the pilonidal sinus leaves little room for doubt concerning its nature. Nevertheless, the possibility exists that it may be a different form of suppurative lesion found in that region. Amongst these, the most important and the most common are the boil and postanal space abscess, which have their origin in the posterior anal crypt. Much more rarely are infected sacrococcygeal teratomas, fibromas, leiomyomas and congenital sinus which originates from the remnants of the spinal canal.

In case of doubt, probing of the tract certainly helps in locating the origin of these lesions which can be confirmed by histological examination of the tissue removed. At times, some atypical cases with shift of the sinuses towards the anus may pose diagnostic dilemma as they might simulate an anal fistula. Nonetheless, the pathognomonic feature is finding of hairs in the sinus and its relationship with an orifice covered by skin which is found along the posterior midline.

Rarely, a pilonidal sinus may extend in the anal canal with clinical features of original disease, but it is wise to exclude the possibility of this being the distal most part of the anal fistula by a thorough examination. An extensive pilonidal sinus tract or abscess may reach up to the anal canal and one has to carefully differentiate the exact origin of the disease process.

Similarly, few atypical forms of fistulas around the anal, ano-coccygeal and sacrococcygeal region may mimic pilonidal sinus disease. These include-

1.   Congenital fistulas of the anal canal- low anal fistulas with an
internal orifice originating from the distal anal canal may have a
squamous epithelial lining. They can be due to the remnants in the
anal and perianal tissue of the ectopic epithelial cells from the
ectodermic proctodial junction and from the post allentoic entodermic
intestine.

2.   Post anal cutaneous dimple- these are formations frequently
found in children, covered with a normal cutaneous epithelium without
hairs. They are attached to the coccyx by means of dense fibrous
bands.

3.   Congenital sinuses derived from the remnants of the spinal
canal - In case of spina bifida, between the spinal canal and the skin
in the sacral region, there may be an orifice secreting CSF which may
get infected to look like a pilonidal sinus, but which can lead to
meningitis if the communication is not closed surgically.

4.   The teratomas and sacrococcygeal dermoid cysts can become
infected and cause abscess and sinuses.

5.   Chronic suppuration of the retro rectal space and of the
sacrococcygeal zone developing after sclerosing therapy for
hemorrhoid, passage of barium through the rectal wall during barium
enema study, osteomyelitis or infections of a benign or malignant
tumor may be mistaken for a pilonidal sinus.

Points to Ponder

   Symptoms related to pilonidal abscess include discomfort or pain,
and intermittent discharge or bleeding. A small group of patients

present with an acute abscess cephalad in the natal cleft. This position distinguishes the disease from other common anorectal problems, such as perirectal abscesses and anal fistulae, which are typically found near the anus. Midline pits are the distinguishing feature, occurring in 100% of cases, and they can typically be identified 4 to 8 cm from the anus. Hair within the abscess cavity is present in approximately two thirds of cases in men and one third of those in women. As the acute abscess resolves, whether spontaneously or with treatment, chronic sinus tracts develop toward the skin.

Further reading and references

1.	Chintapatla S, Safarani N, Kumar S, Haboubi N. Sacrococcygeal pilonidal sinus: historical review, pathological insight and surgical options. Tech Coloproctol. 2003; 7:3-8.

2.	Page BH. The entry of hair into a pilonidal sinus. Br J Surg. 1969; 56:32.

3.	Lee HC, Ho YH, Seow CF, et al. Pilonidal disease in Singapore: clinical features and management. Aust N Z J Surg 2000; 70:196Y8.

4.	Solla JA, Rothenberger DA. Chronic pilonidal disease. An assessment of 150 cases. Dis Colon Rectum 1990; 33:758Y61.

5.	Casberg MA. Infected pilonidal cysts and sinuses. *Bull US Army Med Dept.* 1949; 9:493– 496.

6.	Clothier PR, Haywood IR. The natural history of post anal (pilonidal) sinus. *Ann R Coll Surg Engl.*1984; 66:201–203.

7.	Hanley PH. Symposium: the dilemma of pilonidal disease. Dis Colon Rectum.1977:20:278-298.

8.	Bascom JU. Pilonidal sinus. In: Fazio VW, ed. Current Therapy in Colon and Rectal Surgery. Toronto, Ontario: BC Decker Inc; 1990:32-39.

9.	Allen-Mersh G. Pilonidal sinus: finding the right track for treatment. Br J Surg.1990; 77:123-132.

10.	Nelson JM, Billingham RP. Pilonidal disease and hidradenitis suppurativa. In: Wolff BC, Fleshman JW, Beck DE, Pemberton JH, Wexner SD eds. The ASCRS Textbook of Colon and Rectal Surgery. New York, NY: Springer; 2007:228–239.

Chapter 4

MANAGEMENT OF PILONIDAL SINUS DISEASE

The choice of ideal therapy for pilonidal sinus disease should be guided by several principles, tailored to be patient specific and the gravity of the disease. Regrettably, no single treatment fulfils all these requirements. The projected rate of recurrence and anticipated time to return to work with normal physical activity are important determinants in treatment selection. Both non-operative and operative treatments are efficacious in appropriate settings. Some patients can be treated on an outpatient or day case basis while others require periods in hospital. A sound balance has to be struck between minimizing inpatient treatment without compromising lasting healing.

INVESTIGATING A CASE OF PILONIDAL SINUS DISEASE

MR imaging is able to demonstrate the site and nature of sepsis in patients with pilonidal sinus with the same accuracy as that for fistula in ano. MR imaging can be performed by using a 1.0-T superconducting magnet and body coil, with patients in the supine position. For pilonidal sinus disease, MR imaging can give an approximate sensitivity of 86%, a specificity of 100% a positive predictive value of 100%, and a negative predictive value of 93%. A natal cleft sepsis that reaches the subcutaneous tissues overlying the coccyx and sacrum, and the absence of intersphincteric sepsis or enteric opening, is suggestive of pilonidal sinus disease rather than fistula in ano.

Similarly, a surgeon needs to know the dimensions, location, borders, and branches of the pilonidal sinus cavity in order to plan the operative strategy.

Palpation and methylene blue injection are typically used to estimate the borders of diseased tissue; however, most operative findings do not match the actual borders. Examinations with the use of a 7.5-MHz linear probe on a LOGIQ 5 pro ultrasound scanner, and using power Doppler mode at times, can accurately identify the sinus tract, branches, and its borders. This investigative tool can be employed while deciding upon a surgical intervention for pilonidal sinus patients.

Conservative non-operative management

This is considered for patients without severe symptoms. Conservative therapy is very cost effective because of transfer of treatment from the operating room/inpatient setting to the outpatient clinic. This includes the use of antibiotic therapy to treat infection, avoidance of sepsis and attempts to prevent the need for surgery. Asymptomatic pits do not require treatment.

Meticulous hair control by regular shaving of the natal cleft, removal of hair and scraping of granulation tissue from the sinus is a common practice. However it needs significant time and a long period to achieve results. The protocol requires patient education regarding the nature of the condition and the importance of perineal hygiene. Needless to say that simple lateral incision and drainage of acute abscess, meticulous hair control, and avoiding certain exercises such as sit-ups and leg lifts goes a long way in providing a symptom free period to the patient.

Healing is indicated as an un-inflamed, non-draining natal cleft with shrinkage of the pits.

Role of shaving - Does shaving have a pivotal role in the management of pilonidal sinus disease? Yes, it does control a factor in the disease causation and progression. Hair has three likely pathophysiologic roles: retained hair within a ruptured follicle, secondary invasion through an existing enlarged follicle, and mechanical irritation of pilonidal wounds. Hair in the later two roles maintains the adverse environment within the natal cleft. Hair control addresses these dominant roles and helps the patient focus on perineal hygiene. This, in turn, may prevent follicular plugging with keratin.

Trimming, shaving, and plucking are the ways to get rid of the hair. However, many patients find this important phase of treatment as clumsy, inconvenient and difficult.

Although simple, shaving requires the same attention to detail as any operation. Adequate exposure and lighting of the natal cleft are essential to ensure complete shaving of all hair within the natal cleft, 5 cm from the anus to the pre and parasacral area. One should not miss even the thin and fine hairs. All the visible hair within the sinus should be picked up without attempting to probe and extract hair within the sinus. Performing the initial shave may need 5 or more minutes, but the subsequent shaves will take half of this time. The end points of shaving are disappearance of patient symptoms and resolution of acute inflammation and discharge.

The shaving should be continued if the pits look drier and smaller at each shave. Patient education is critical for successful outcome. Once educated, the patient can manage this maneuver well and can sense symptoms of recurrence, when he resumes weekly shaving and improves his perineal hygiene. Family members can be easily trained to assist the patient in managing recurrence. The average patient requires three to four shavings per episode, with a range from two to eight.

Antibiotics

Bacterial colonization of pilonidal sinuses has historically ranged from 50 to 70%, typical isolates including Staphylococcus aureus and anaerobes such as Bacteroides. Anaerobes can be isolated in 52% at initial presentation and 64% in recurrent conditions. However, two randomized trials have failed to demonstrate any significant improvement in wound healing with an empirical course of antibiotics. Having previously shown an association between anaerobic infection and delay in healing of granulating wounds, studies have suggested that there is no role for empirical antibiotics in the conservative management of pilonidal disease and that antibiotics should be reserved for patients with clinical evidence of infection.

A new classification of the disease is proposed based on the concept of the 'navicular area'. The navicular area defines the extent of the natal cleft described by its lateral edges and posterior extent. The patient is placed in the jack-knife position. When the buttocks are pushed together, the outer lines of contact represent the lateral edges of the natal cleft. Its inferior extent is the posterior border of the anal triangle, which has its tip at the apex of the coccyx and its base between the ischial tuberosities. The edges are marked with a pen prior to releasing the buttocks and a ship-like shape is revealed, referred to as the 'navicular area' (Fig.1).

Classification with reference to the navicular area may be useful in taking decision about the treatment in sacrococcygeal pilonidal sinus disease.

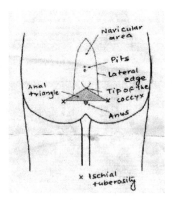

Figure 1- The navicular area

A classification of the disease into five types is proposed.

Type I: Asymptomatic pit(s) without a history of abscess and/or drainage. The pits are almost always within the navicular area and require no surgical therapy. Regular local hair removal and good personal hygiene is all what is needed in this situation.

Type II: Acute pilonidal abscess. The treatment is always drainage using a lateral incision. They may require further surgical treatment after resolution of the acute symptoms.

Type III: Pit(s) within the navicular area with a history of abscess and/or previous drainage. Different conservative or minimal surgical approaches usually suffice.

Type IV: Extensive disease where one or more sinus opening lies outside the navicular area. Such patients usually have a history of multiple abscess formation and drainages without definitive pilonidal surgery. A more aggressive surgical approach is required in such situation.

Type V: Recurrent pilonidal sinus following any surgical treatment. A flap or plastic procedure together with an attempt to flatten the natal cleft may be needed.

EXPERIMENTAL TREATMENTS

These are considered for patients without severe symptoms. Looking at the diversified presentation of the disease, lack of unanimity towards a gold standard of treatment, varied results of the conventional approaches within different institutions, few experimental procedures have emerged in the treatment of this disease complex. While they have been used with some success in the experienced hands, they have been a disappointment for others. However, a fair trial of such treatment options can be given as an attempt to prevent the need for surgery.

Phenol

Phenol injection therapy (phenolization) was first described by Maurice and Greenwood in 1964. They suggested that it might supply a cure to the quiescent phase in the treatment of PSD. They suggested using phenol at 80% concentration or in its crystallized form (The crystallized phenol turns into liquid form at body temperature and fill the sinus). This concentration of phenol solution or the crystallized form was observed to cause destruction in the pilonidal sinus cavities, together with narrowing of the lipoid tissue, sacral fascia and skin.

This method was chosen to avoid excision of the sinuses and it was based on the destruction of the pathologic epithelium of the sinus. Pioneers of the method thought that if the epithelium of the tract could be destroyed, any infection present sterilized and if all the embedded hair in the tracts removed, then the sinus should heal.

Phenol injection can be given on an inpatient or on an outpatient basis. Ideally, the injection should be done at a quiescent phase and a pre injection course of an appropriate antibiotic may be useful in some cases. Most researchers advocating the use of phenol have reported a success rate between 59% and 95.1% for the treatment, a repeat rate of 6.3% to 17.1%, and median healing times of 6.2 to 8.7 weeks. Work days lost are reported as 8.3–11.6 days.

Procedure of phenol injection- The patient is placed in a prone jack knife position. After shaving of the sacral area, the buttocks are held apart with 7-5 cm strapping to expose the sacral area and anal verge. The skin of the area is cleansed with an antiseptic solution and then dried and toweled up in the usual manner. The skin around the sinus is protected by liberal smearing of Vaseline while protecting the anus with Vaseline gauze. By a gentle probing, any loose hairs present are removed with forceps from the sinus and from the side tracts. The main sinus tract is then injected with a solution of 80% phenol using a blunt nosed needle which can fit into the sinus opening snugly or by introducing an infant feeding tube in the tract. Using minimum of pressure, the solution is then injected in the tract taking care to avoid phenol being forced into the tissue surrounding the sinus and causing a local inflammatory reaction (Fig.2).

The injection is stopped when phenol is seen coming from any of the openings and any excess is quickly wiped away. The solution is allowed to remain in the tract for one minute, after which firm pressure is applied around the sinus tract to express the phenol and to bring out loose hairs to the surface, which can be picked out. The whole procedure is repeated twice, each time leaving the phenol in situ for one minute, thereby giving a total exposure time of three minutes. The whole tract is then washed out with saline and curetted. Vaseline gauze and a light dressing are applied to the injected area. The patients are instructed to have frequent baths. Strict hygiene of the area is emphasized during the healing period. After the sinuses have healed, it is advisable to wash the natal cleft after defecation rather than using toilet paper. Special care must be taken to dust off the loose hairs, particularly after a visit to the barber.

Another study has found even better results using 40% phenol solution on an outpatient basis.

The most common postoperative complications after phenol treatment are sterile abscesses and fat and skin necrosis which have been reported in about 7–16% of patients and is ascribed to leakage of phenol into the surrounding tissues either due to too much pressure at the time of injection, or due to opening up of a false tract during preliminary probing.

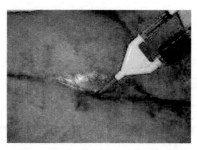

Figure 2- Phenolization of the sinus tract

Use of Polyphenols- Humic substances or natural polyphenols are natural liquid biopolymers which are the by-products of soil organic matter degradation and are present in the environment. Humic substances have been in use in balneotherapy for a long time and a similar hypothesis has been applied to use polyphenols in the treatment of pilonidal sinus disease.

Polyphenols are known to remove microorganisms located in the wound bed. They can cover and fill infected cavities, which in turn prevent atmospheric oxygen from reaching the microorganisms. Polyphenols can also prevent the microorganisms from using oxygen present in blood and neighboring tissues produced due to their antioxidant actions.

Polyphenols have been claimed to increase the chemotaxis of phagocytes to the diseased area. Additionally they can enhance the capacity of granulocytes to engulf bacteria. Polyphenols also increase the activities of lysosomal enzymes which are transferred into the phagolysosomes and lyse bacteria. Polyphenols are known to promote wound healing also.

Polyphenols have been proposed to promote cytokine, interferon and tumor necrosis factor alpha (TNF-α) synthesis for faster healing. This in turn exerts anti-inflammatory actions and causes the wound healing process to proceed better. Theoretically, healthy fibrin formation and collagen synthesis result in better wound healing and consequently in better healing of the sinuses.

Taking into consideration all the above factors, Sodium humate 25% was used as the source of polyphenol in one study. Three polyphenol product forms (Pilonol®) were used altogether to achieve best results.

The area under treatment was first depilated and a teaspoon full of Pilonol solution was poured onto the affected region and was massaged for two to three minutes at bed time and was covered with a gauze which was left in place until next morning when the previous application was washed out by the Pilonol gel®. This was followed by application of Pilonol cream®. The treatment continued till complete healing was achieved. Following the treatment, patients were advised to obey general personal hygiene rules, to have frequent baths while keeping the sacrococcygeal region depilated for at least one year. The study claimed a fair outcome of this conservative treatment for pilonidal sinus.

The major disadvantage of topical polyphenol treatment is the need for regular applications for a pretty long time, which look to be cumbersome and unbearable to many of the patients. Few patients also experienced local reactions in the form of irritation, erythema, burning and aching sensation.

Laser epilation- As it is known that the hair follicles are involved with recurrent bacterial infection in pilonidal sinus disease; various methods of hair removal with different light sources have emerged. Similarly, a pilonidal sinus usually contains hair and extensive vascularization due to inflammation, which theoretically gives laser, waves the potential to destroy the deep fistula systems of the sinus without affecting the overlying skin.

It was postulated that permanent destruction of the hair follicles of a certain area can be achieved by transmitting heat to the target hair. Progressive hair destruction is possible to achieve using laser treatments, resulting in hair reduction for years of follow-up. In one study, patients were treated with laser epilation using an alexandrite laser (GentleLase, Candela, Wayland, MA, USA) or with an intense pulsed light device (Epilight, Lumenis, Santa Clara, CA, USA). Hairs were removed in a round area 4 to 5 cm around the affected area. Treatments were performed at 6- to 8-week intervals for the first three to four sittings and then at every 8 to 16 weeks until remission of infection and removal of most of the hair were achieved. It is also claimed that in patients with recurrent folliculitis, natal cleft laser hair removal resolved the folliculitis and prevented future surgery.

The laser treatment is however, not cost effective and has not been favored by many because of the lengthy duration involved.

Thread dragging and pad pressure therapy- This is one of the traditional Chinese medicine therapy used for complex fistulas and sinuses. In this procedure, the sinus tract is curetted free of all the debris and hairs. Ten threads are inserted from one end of the sinus tract to emerge from the other and tied. Each day, the part of the threads lying within the tract are pulled outside and cleaned with saline till the size of the wound is reduced and dragging of the thread becomes difficult. Five of the threads are then removed and remaining five are left behind until the wound gets reduced further and no more discharge is found (Fig.3). This is followed by application of a pad over the wound with a pressure strapping to accelerate wound healing. This procedure was claimed to have a successful outcome.

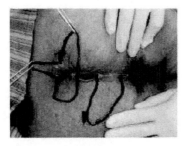

Figure 3- Thread dragging of sinuses

Fibrin glue- In the recent time, treatment of an epithelized track like the fistula-in-ano has been obliterated with a reasonable success using fibrin tissue glue. The advantage of using fibrin glue to treat fistula-in-ano is that healing of the track can be achieved without excision of a large amount of tissue and without disruption to the sphincter complex. Fibrin glue has also been used as an adjunct to reduce postoperative infection in primary wound closure after wide excision of the pilonidal sinus complex.

In one of the pilot study, plugging the sinus tract with fibrin glue was performed as the sole treatment for pilonidal sinus. The pilonidal pits were identified under general anesthesia and all the debris were removed from the pits. The sinus tracks were thoroughly curetted or brushed through the midline pits with a small Volkmann's spoon or cytology brush to remove the epithelium of the sinus. The pits were then injected with fibrin glue (Tisseel®, Baxter Healthcare Ltd, Newbury, UK). One to 2 ml of glue was injected into the sinus complex to occlude as much of the sinus complex as possible (Fig.4).This was done as an outpatient treatment with a regular follow-up. Five of the six patients treated with this technique had their sinuses healed.

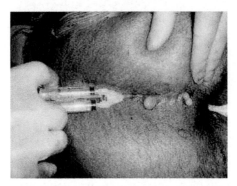

Figure 4- Injection of fibrin glue in the sinus tract

POINTS TO PONDER

Conservative treatments for PD have gained popularity because of the high morbidity associated with the surgical procedures of PD. Conservative non-operative treatment for PD constitutes meticulous hair control by shaving the natal cleft, better perineal hygiene, various experimental procedures described above and at times, limited lateral incision and drainage of acute abscesses. Implementation of the conservative treatment strategy has resulted in a substantial decrease in the admission rates of PD patients in the hospitals.

The efficacy and failure rate varies between institutions and the surgeons and the most optimal type of conservative treatment is required to be tailored to suit the individual patient.

A proportion of patients who are not suitable for conservative measures or who have severe, worsening, or recurrent disease, should be offered a surgical reconstructive procedure by a surgeon familiar with these techniques.

Further reading and references

1.   Armstrong JH, Barcia PJ. Pilonidal sinus disease: the conservative approach. Arch Surg. 1994; 129:914 –918.

2.   Karydakis GE. Easy and successful treatment of pilonidal sinus after explanation of its causative process. ANZ J Surg. 1992; 62:385–389.

3.   Tezel E. A new classification according to navicular area concept for sacrococcygeal pilonidal disease. Colorectal Disease.2007; 9: 572–576.

4.   Conroy FJ, Kandamany N, Mahaffey PJ. Laser depilation and hygiene: preventing recurrent pilonidal sinus disease. *J Plast Reconstr Aesthet Surg.* 2008; 61:1069 –1072.

5.   Jensen SL, Harling H. Prognosis after simple incision and drainage for a first episode acute pilonidal abscess. Br J Surg. 1988; 75:60-61.

6.   Kayaalp C, Aydin C. Review of phenol treatment in sacrococcygeal pilonidal disease. *Tech Coloproctol* 2009; 13:189 – 193.

7.   Aksoy HM, Aksoy B, Egemen D. Effectiveness of topical use of natural polyphenons for the treatment of sacrococcygeal pilonidal sinus disease: a retrospective study including 192 patients. Eur J Dermatol. 2010; 20:476-81.

8.   Kitchen P. Pilonidal sinus - management in the primary care setting. Aust Fam Physician 2010; 39:372–375.

9.   Humphries AE, Duncan JE. Evaluation and management of pilonidal disease. Surg Clin North Am 2010; 90:113–124.

10.   Bascom J. Pilonidal disease: origin from follicles of hairs and results of follicle removal as treatment. Surgery 1980; 87:567–72.

11.   Lu JG, Wang C, Cao YQ, Yao YB. Thread-dragging and pad pressure therapy in traditional Chinese medicine for treatment of pilonidal sinus: a case report. Zhong Xi Yi Jie He Xue Bao. 2011; 9:36-7.

12.   Handmer M. Sticking to the facts: a systematic review of fibrin glue for pilonidal disease.ANZ J Surg. 2012; 82:221-4.

Chapter 5

SURGICAL TREATMENT OF PILONIDAL SINUS DISEASE

While management of Pilonidal Sinus Disease still remains controversial and debatable, surgical intervention does hold field as the main mode of treatment. Although no single approach or surgical technique can be relied upon to minimize morbidity and prevent the recurrence, it is in general remains the ultimate choice by most of the surgeons. Many surgical procedures that are available for symptomatic PSD range from simple shaving and opening of the sinus tracts to complex flap repairs. However, none of these alone is perfect in providing quicker wound healing, non-recurrence outcome and abolition of sepsis. The choice of a particular surgical approach depends on the surgeon's familiarity with the procedure and perceived result in terms of preventing recurrence of sinus and a quick healing of resulting cavity or surgical wound.

Acute Pilonidal Abscess

Most patients present initially with pain, tenderness, swelling, and erythema in the gluteal cleft with or without drainage from the involved area (Fig.1). Primary pits may be visible in the midline of the gluteal cleft; however, they are often obscured.

For acute abscesses, various treatment options are available:

- *Aspiration* followed by treatment with antibiotics and later curative intent surgery.

- *Drainage without curettage:* simple drainage of abscess.

- *Drainage and curettage:* surgical drainage of abscess and curettage of cavity to remove hair and granulation tissue.

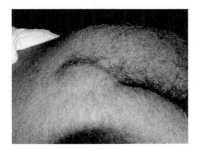

Figure 1- Acute pilonidal abscess

Of these choices, draining the abscess followed by curettage of the cavity has the advantage of quick relief of symptoms and early return to work in all cases. Incision and drainage is recommended as the first treatment because it is a simple office procedure performed under local anesthesia and offers relief of symptoms followed by a quick recovery.

A technique which involved needle aspiration of the abscess with consecutive slow injections of equal amount of local anesthetic into the abscess cavity via the same needle to provide analgesia to be followed by incision and a gentle curettage of the cavity was found to be very effective. This method seems to eliminate multiple infiltrations of the abscess cavity and the surrounding area with the anesthetic, obviating the associated pain of such injections.

In another study, unroofing and curettage was found associated with higher rate of healing and lower rate of recurrence when compared with mere incision and drainage of the abscess. Complete healing could be achieved in more than half of the patients. Recurrence occurred in 25% of those with initial healing and the overall cure rate at 18 months was around 75%. Bascom advocated placing a lateral incision 2.5 cm away from the midline and cutting adequate button of skin to prevent premature resealing.

The patients who are more likely to experience failure or recurrence are predicted by significantly more midline pits and lateral sinus tracts. A lateral incision should be preferred so that midline pits do not interfere with healing of the wound. The cavity should also be vigorously curetted, debriding the walls off embedded hairs and a meticulously depilated surrounding skin not only at the time of operation, but also over subsequent weeks. The value of using methylene blue to identify associated sinus tracts is variable. Some authors note that it does not completely diffuse through the tracts due to their blockage with semisolid material which obstructs the path of the dye. Another author cited the unreliability of marking dyes that resulted in overaggressive resection of affected tissues. He accused frequent recurrences to overreliance on the dye which at time stain the non existing tracts and the tissues around.

CHRONIC OR RECURRENT PILONIDAL SINUS DISEASE

For chronic and recurrent sinuses, various techniques have been reported. The choice of a particular surgical approach is dependent on the surgeon's familiarity with the procedure and perceived results in terms of low recurrence of sinus and of quick healing of resulting cavity or surgical wound.

The ideal treatment for a pilonidal sinus disease should be simple to perform with limited inpatient stay. It should cause minimal postoperative pain and need limited wound care to provide early return to activity. While having a low recurrence rate, it should also be cost effective. However, none of the available procedures fulfils all these criteria and therefore the one which is most suited to the particular patient's disease condition should be chosen.

For chronic or recurrent pilonidal sinuses, excision of all involved skin and subcutaneous tissue may be necessary for definitive treatment. The resultant wounds may then either be left open to heal by secondary intention, or may be closed by primary suture. Advocates of open technique state that reduced wound tension facilitates trouble free healing without recurrence if all sinus tracts are fully excised. The open approach has the advantage of brief hospitalization, but substantial morbidity results from a prolonged healing and the need of frequent, uncomfortable dressing changes. For the patients who are typically young, otherwise healthy, and active, these wounds cause considerable social and economic disability on account of reduced mobility and action.

The simpler procedures- 'less is more'-
The easiest procedure to deal with pilonidal sinuses is laying open the tract. This was originally described by Buie in 1938. With this technique the surgeon simply unroofs the midline and lateral sinus tracts, which are then allowed to heal by secondary intention.

Laying open of track (Pilonidal sinotomy)

The procedure is carried out under local anesthesia with the patient in a jack knife position. After shaving off the hairs around the sinuses and cleaning the area with Povidone Iodine, the skin and the subcutaneous tissue is infiltrated with 5-12 ml of a solution of 2% Xylocain and Adrenalin [1:200000].

Methylene blue dye mixed with hydrogen peroxide is injected in one of the external opening to give a guideline about the tract and branching. An anal fistula probe is inserted in the tract and tract is laid open over the length of the probe. When two or more sinus openings are found joining each other, the fistula tract and the skin between them is incised (Fig.2).

Any hairs and foreign material if found, are removed. All the tracts are traced and the infected and indurated tissue is scooped out, leaving behind a red, raw area. No attempt is made to deepen the dissection up to the post sacral fascia and a layer of tissue is left between the floor of the wound and the sacrum & coccyx. Care is taken that the wound should acquire a shape of an inverted cone, wide externally and narrows internally. This prevents premature closure of the external skin wound.

The wound is tucked with paraffin gauze and is then covered with a padded adhesive dressing.

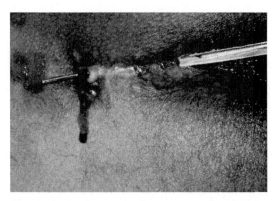

Figure 2- Laying open the tract over a probe

Lord and Millar proposed a closed technique in which the sinus tracts are not opened up but instead debrided with a "bottle" brush. They also recognized the importance of the tiny midline pits in the pathogenesis of the disease and excised them down to the cavity, effectively unroofing them. It is a simple operation that can be done under local anesthesia as an outpatient procedure.

The procedure - Using local infiltration of I per cent xylocaine with adrenaline, the pits are excised down to the underlying cavity and track through a small elliptical incision. The aim is to remove as little normal skin as possible, not more than half centimeters to each side of the midline. No attempt is made to remove the cavity as this is lined with granulation tissue. The cavity is deroofed to drain freely. Any hairs within it are picked out with forceps and the cavity mopped clean. All the hairs in the cavity are removed with the help the tiny 'bottle' brush with nylon bristles such as is used for cleaning electric razors. The lesion heals faster if all the hairs can be removed, including those lurking in lateral or midline tracks.

The track is stretched with sinus forceps. The brush is then inserted and rotated. Hairs become entangled in the bristles of the brush and are easily seen when the brush is withdrawn. This is repeated several times until there is no more hair. At times, a hydrogen peroxide washout can help loosen the hairs and clean out the cavity and track. It is essential that the track drains freely both ways-onto the surface and into the cavity. It is sometimes wise to excise a tiny disk of skin from around a lateral opening to help ensure good drainage.

A meticulous shaving for a centimeter around the edge of the excision wound is an integral part of the treatment, and this is repeated at 2- or 3-week intervals until healing is complete.

A general shave of the whole area is desirable for reasons of hygiene and also because strapping is used to hold the dressing in position. It is, of course, well recognized that shaving alone may allow some pilonidal sinuses to heal. The patient is sent home with a large gauze pack held in place by strapping.

Reported recurrence rates in this technique however, vary widely between 6.5% and 40.5%.

The importance of avoiding midline incisions and placing any healing wounds off midline to reduce recurrence was recognized by Bascom. In Bascom's procedure, a lateral incision is made over the sinus cavity, which is curetted to remove hair and granulation tissue. The incision is left open with a light dressing to heal by secondary intention. He excised the midline pits and sinus tracts rather than

simply brushing the sinus tracts as in Lord and Millar's procedure
(Fig.3).

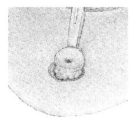

Figure 3- Pit excision

Another minimally invasive technique describes an ambulatory
surgical treatment for pilonidal disease which integrates the principles
suggested by both Lord and Millar and Bascom by introducing the
use of skin trephines, for the excision of pilonidal pits and
debridement of underlying cavities and tracts (Fig.4).

The procedure is performed under local anesthesia. All openings
and tracts are cored out utilizing Keyes skin trephines, 2.0 to 9.0 mm
in diameter. Small pits with short tracts are removed with smaller
trephines. Pits leading to subcutaneous cavities are then excised
down to the cavity with mid-sized trephines. Openings of fistulas and
drainage openings for acute suppurations needs excision using large
trephines.

For each opening, the trephine is inserted perpendicularly to the
skin. After penetrating the skin, the trephine is aligned in the direction
of the tract and excision is continued until the pilonidal cavity is
entered, thus removing all epithelized openings and scarred fistulous

tracts. Individual pits can be easily removed with just one hand twist and with minimal rims of tissue not exceeding 1.0 to 2.0 mm. Curved forceps and a bone curette are then introduced through the openings to thoroughly clean all cavities and tracts from hair, debris, and granulation tissue. Trephines can also be used as chisels within the cavity, to carve out scar tissue and embedded hair. All these openings are left unpacked without suturing. Patients are kept supine under an hour-long observation before discharge.

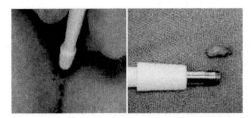

Figure 4- pit excision using trephines

The rationale given behind using trephines is that when inserted through pit openings, trephines serve as sharp debridement tools within pilonidal cavities and along fistulous tracts thus obviating the use of brushes. The round opening produced by the trephine serves as a drainage port, providing undisturbed continued outflow of infected fluid until the pilonidal cavity dries and collapses from within, thus making the use of drains or extensive incisions unnecessary. By individually punching out each pit, gaps of unaffected healthy skin are left to link and hold the opposed sides of the natal cleft. These bridges stabilize the perforated roof of the pilonidal cavity, prevent lateral traction of cavity walls and skin margins, and facilitate undistorted healing of the natal cleft with minimal scarring.

In a large numbered study of about 1100 patients, the overall recurrence rate reported was 16 percent, thus showing the usefulness of this simple procedure.

UNROOFING AND OPEN SECONDARY HEALING

Excision of midline tracts followed by an open wound leads to prolonged healing. Unroofing of the tracts minimizes the midline wound and shortens healing time accordingly. This approach is effective in the presence of a concomitant abscess. Recurrence has been reported to be less than 13% with this technique. A dye like methylene blue is instilled into the pilonidal sinus and an elliptical excision is made to include a margin of healthy tissue along with the tract and cavity down to the sacral/gluteal fascia (Fig.5). The resultant cavity is then packed with a moist dressing and left to heal by second intention. The dressings need to be changed at regular intervals and the patient is seen by a surgeon once a week in the outpatient clinic.

Autologous platelet-rich plasma (PRP) gel consists of cytokines, growth factors, chemokines, and a fibrin scaffold derived from a patient's blood, all of which mediate wound healing. The mechanism of action for PRP gel is thought to be the molecular and cellular induction of normal wound healing responses similar to that seen with platelet activation. This therapy is used in hard-to-heal acute and chronic wounds. One study prospectively investigated 52 patients who underwent excisional therapy of pilonidal sinuses with open secondary healing. Patients were randomized to platelet concentrate thrombin mixture applied to the wound or no therapy. Wound healing rates were 24 versus 30 days in favor of the treated group. Improved quality of life and earlier return to activity were also noted in this treatment group. PRP gel was found to have a positive impact on wound healing and associated factors such as pain and infection in such large wounds.

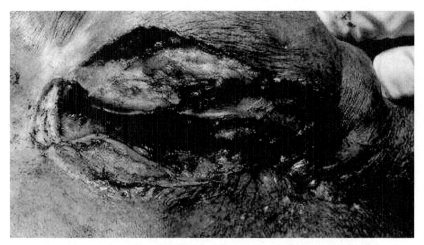

Figure 5- Wide excision with healing by secondary intention

Some workers have used a medicated seton technique, whereas the thread impregnated with medication having both cutting as well as healing properties was inserted in the tract and was gradually tied to induce pressure necrosis as well as simultaneous healing ending into a healed wound without the need of anesthesia or hospitalization. A single cutting seton (garrote) can also be applied in an ambulatory care setting under local anesthesia. It is tied and progressively tightened over a period of few weeks. This leads to excision of the diseased area with revascularization of the wounds site and healing by secondary intention, leaving an acceptable scar.

More recently, negative pressure dressings, which promote granulation, have been suggested as an alternative to open packing. Primary VAC therapy (V.A.C. Therapy1, Kinetic Concepts, San Antonio, TX) following excision of pilonidal sinus has been reported with favorable results. It may be performed as an outpatient procedure with low risk of primary failure or infection while accelerating healing and reducing the frequency of dressing changes.

In randomized controlled trials compared with wet-to-dry dressing changes, VAC therapy has demonstrated significantly faster healing of chronic wounds. Negative pressure exerted on wounds has been shown to increase local blood flow, up regulate cell proliferation, decrease bacterial counts, and facilitate wound granulation. The benefits of negative pressure wound therapy should be applicable to pilonidal disease and early reports are encouraging; however, follow-up for recurrence has not been reported.

INCISION WITH MARSUPIALIZATION

Marsupialization is defined as suturing the skin edges, whether to the postsacral fascia or to the subcutaneous tissue after excision.

This approach involves opening the sinus tracts in the midline to include all the secondary tracts. The posterior and lateral fibrous tissue is then left in situ and sutured to the skin edge or dermis. The goal is to reduce the effective wound healing area thus reducing the time of healing. During the marsupialization procedure, the sinus floor is left undissected, and the boundary of the fibrous floor of the sinus cavity is used to suture the skin edges. This prevents suture tension, and because the fibrous tissue does not contain free nerve endings, it may result in less pain, eventually leading to the quicker return to work.

Several studies have evaluated the effectiveness of incision with marsupialization when compared with excisional therapy. Karayakalli concluded that although healing time and postoperative care was longer in patients with marsupialization, other factors such as quality of life, return to work time, and pain scores were favored in unroofing and marsupialization when compared with excisional therapy followed by flap closure.

The Procedure- A grooved director or mosquito clamp is inserted into the sinus opening .The tract is opened throughout its extent into normal appearing fatty tissue in order to ensure an adequate opening of the tract. All friable granulation tissue and hair are removed by wiping with gauze. A search is then made with a probe for additional openings at the base and sides. The overhanging skin edges are undermined for a short distance and separated from the tract. Occasionally this will demonstrate extension of a sinus which might have overlooked. The skin surrounding a sinus opening is excised; Allis forceps are applied to the edges of the cavity, and a wedge removed by sharp dissection. Only a small portion of the cavity is left behind. After achieving hemostasis, the skin is sutured to the edge of the remaining cavity with single interrupted 2/0 chromic sutures. The ends of the sutures are left long so that if the sutures cut through, they can be easily grasped and removed. By undercutting the skin and removing a large wedge of cavity, the process of healing is definitely hastened (Fig.6).

Postoperatively, the wound is covered with antiseptic tulle for a couple of days, and subsequently with a dry dressing and is left to secondary healing. Weekly inspection of the wound is essential, when patients are instructed about wound care together with a shower twice a day.

The advocates of this procedure believe that shorter hospital stay, earlier return to work or school, lower levels of self-reported pain, and lower rates of complications are the main advantages of unroofing and marsupialization. However, potential inconvenience of wound care and longer healing time after this surgical technique are the major deterrents.

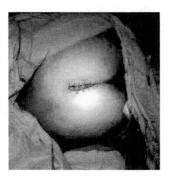

Figure 6- Marsupialization after tract excision

BASCOM CHRONIC ABSCESS CURETTAGE WITH MIDLINE PIT
EXCISION (PIT PICKING SURGERY, BASCOM I)

Bascom designed an operation based on the hypothesis that the hair follicle itself, not the hair shaft, was the source of local sepsis. Midline pits are conservatively excised with removal of contiguous hair and debris in the pits. The use of trephines and disposable dermatologic punch biopsy instruments (2–3 mm) is an excellent method to excise the infected, epithelized sinus pit, while still minimizing the extent of the midline wound. A concomitant lateral incision, parallel to the midline wound, is made to curette the debris from the cavity connecting the sinus pits. All incisions are usually left open to heal by secondary intention.

The procedure is also useful in dealing with acute abscess. The abscess is drained and allowed to subside before the follicle removal is attempted. The drainage incisions are kept on the lateral aspect of the midline. Once the wound become dry, the follicles are removed from the lateral incisions as they are easily visible in the midline wound from where the drainage was done. Wounds are followed closely to remove hair that may gravitate into the wound. Careful and frequent wound care is essential for the success of this technique. This care is optimally provided in an office equipped with proper lighting and a proctoscopic table for optimal exposure. However, reliance upon visiting nurses or family members to provide wound care is unsatisfactory.

SINUS EXCISION AND PRIMARY CLOSURE

The sinus, including all extensions, is radically excised. If guiding is needed, methylene blue dye can be injected. The excision includes all extensions and diseased tissue and is performed with sharp dissection by use of scissors or diathermy. The wounds are closed in layers supplemented with mass sutures with as little tension as possible. Absorbable interrupted sutures are used to close the subcutaneous fascia (Fig.7). The mass sutures encompassing fascia, subcutis, and skin are tied over gauze packs to avoid dead space. No flaps or a deliberate attempt for off-midline closures is used. The mass sutures are removed after 5 to 7 days and the skin sutures after 2 weeks. It has been observed that midline closure procedures offer a quicker healing time but have high rates of recurrence and failure of primary healing.

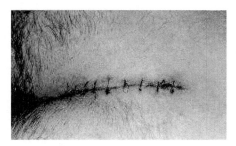

Figure 7-Midline closure after excision of the tract

A 'D' shaped excision followed by closure with suction drain is being proposed which can be performed under local anesthesia as a day care surgery with acceptable outcome. Obeid proposed a technique of en-block excision of sinus area followed by primary suturing which, while sounding interesting, did not found much favor by others.

An interesting study was conducted to try to improve upon existing conservative techniques in the treatment of chronic pilonidal sinus by using human dermal tissue allograft. A prospective study of 46 consecutive patients undergoing 47 operations for pilonidal disease was conducted by three surgeons. All patients underwent a conservative surgical technique with injection of human dermal tissue allograft and primary wound closure on an ambulatory basis. Sixty percent of patients required no postoperative narcotic use. Eighty-five percent missed no work or school. Sixty-six percent healed primarily. Thirty-three percent of patients developed minor wound complications that quickly responded to suture removal and drainage. There were no wound failures. The recurrence rate was 11% with a median follow-up of 15 months.

SEVERE AND RECURRENT DISEASE

Despite well-intended and frequently performed conservative approaches to control initial disease, recurrent infections remain a serious problem. Infrequently, patients develop complex pilonidal disease, which is characterized by chronic or recurrent abscesses and extensive, branching sinus tracts. This manifestation of the disease demands a more aggressive surgical approach, and definitive treatment requires wide excision of all involved tissue. Primary closure of these wounds is not a viable option given a dehiscence rate of up to 37%, and open management with healing by secondary intention is not suitable because of the length of time that would be required for healing. Reconstructive procedures are typically required in these cases. These procedures not only cover the wound but also, in theory, flatten the natal cleft, reducing hair accumulation, mechanical irritation, and risk of recurrence. Each offers relatively short healing time but requires an extensive operation and prolonged hospitalization. Complications, including flap necrosis, wound dehiscence, and infections pose major challenge.

Evidence continues to support flap closure off the midline, particularly as to reducing the time of healing. But some authors have questioned the value of such techniques, arguing that flaps are technically more demanding than open-wound procedures and that they increase rates of loss of skin sensation. These authors suggest limiting their use to recurrent or complex pilonidal sinuses only. The following pages include a brief summary of commonly performed flap procedures.

KARYDAKIS FLAP

Karydakis was the first to advocate asymmetric closure of pilonidal wounds to decrease recurrence. This technique avoids placing a wound in the midline at the depth of the natal cleft. It also flattens the cleft, reducing hair accumulation and mechanical irritation. In this advancing flap operation, an asymmetric elliptical incision is made around all involved tissue down to the postsacral fascia and the wound is undermined, creating a thick flap that is closed off midline. The procedure- Under general anesthesia, with the patient in the prone position, the buttocks taped apart. A line is drawn 2 cm paramedian to the natal cleft; this line is placed on the same side as any lateral secondary opening or scar. If the sinuses are entirely central, either side is chosen. The pilonidal cavity is probed and its longitudinal and lateral limits are marked. Using the initial paramedian line as its longitudinal axis, an ellipse is drawn that included the entire pilonidal cavity. The caudal tip of the ellipse is placed a further 1 cm laterally (i.e., 3 cm lateral to the midline) to avoid the final wound curving toward the anus. The edge of the ellipse is infiltrated with 20 ml of 1 percent lidocaine hydrochloride with adrenaline 1 in 200,000. The medial edge of the ellipse is incised with a scalpel perpendicular to the skin and down to, but not through, the thoracolumbar fascia overlying the sacrum. The ellipse's lateral border is incised at an angle of 45° to the skin to meet the medial incision, thus removing the ellipse of tissue. Although the length of the ellipse itself may vary, it is usually 8- to 10-cm long. The lateral edge of the ellipse is made exactly symmetrical with the medial edge, which usually led to excising more skin and fat well beyond the sinuses. The temptation to reduce the size of the ellipse by reducing the concavity of the lateral edge of the ellipse is strongly resisted to avoid producing a vertical suture line that is in the midline and not on its side. In such fashion, the width of the ellipse is usually at least 4 to 6 cm. Only skin incision is made with a scalpel while the diathermy is used to remove the ellipse, including all sinuses and secondary openings down to the muscle and sacral fascia. Extreme caution is practiced to avoid inadvertent contamination of the wound by opening the track of the sinus or its ramifications. The specimen is inspected to ensure complete excision of the sinus complex and then it is sent for histological examination.

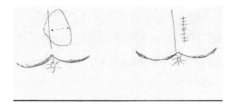

Figure 8- Karydaki's technique

Hemostasis is secured and a suction drain is brought out lateral to the wound. A 1-cm thick, 2-cm wide flap is mobilized with cutting diathermy along the entire medial edge of the wound. In patients whose disease is close to the anus, particular care is taken to avoid trauma to the sphincters. Interrupted 2.0 sutures are placed at 1-cm intervals between the deep limit of the medial flap and the longitudinal midline of the base of the elliptical cavity; the buttock tapes are released and the sutures tied. A second layer of interrupted 2.0 is placed at 1-cm intervals between the free edge of the medial flap and the lateral aspect of the wound (Fig.8). The skin is closed with subcuticular stitches and a light dressing is applied to the closed wound. Patients are nursed in the prone or lateral positions. Walking is not restricted. Patients are discharged on the second postoperative day after being taught to estimate the daily effluent of the suction drain. The suction drain is removed when the effluent is less than 50 ml per 24 hours for two consecutive days, which usually occurs around the tenth postoperative day. Sutures are also removed along with the suction drain, and patients are allowed to return to work by the third postoperative week.

In the Karydakis series, less than 1% of over 5000 patients, followed over 20 years, developed recurrence. The wound complication rate approximated 9%.

BASCOM CLEFT LIFT (BASCOM II)

Bascom cleft lift closure involves excision of the unhealed skin and sinus tracts. A full thickness skin flap is mobilized across the gluteal cleft to create an off-midline closure. The goal of this procedure is to completely eliminate the gluteal cleft in the diseased area. The gluteal fat is allowed to appose and excess skin is excised to re-contour the natal cleft and allow a shallower closure away from the midline. Its main differences, when compared with the Karydakis flap, are the lack of excision and mobilization of the fatty subcutaneous tissues and the reliance upon skin flaps.

The procedure- Midline pits and lateral openings are probed, and the gluteal side containing the most lateral sinus or the side to which the lateral tracts extended i.e., the most affected buttock side is identified. If this happened to be the left side, an asymmetric ellipse-like incision is performed mostly on the left side to create a spindle-shaped island of skin, which also involved the midline pits. The apex of the incision is extended superior and left lateral to the top of the gluteal cleft in such a way that its left border coincided with the ipsilateral line of buttocks contact. In this way, the amount of skin involved on the left side is twice the natural depth of the midgluteal cleft.

The incision crosses the midline to the right at an acute angle superior to the most cephalad extension of the sinus (as that is defined by initial probing of the midline pits) and at a right angle inferior to the lower portion of the pilonidal cyst back to the left side. There, it became comma-shaped, pointing toward the anus and thus creating the inferior corner of the wound. Thus, both corners lay to the left of the midline. The incision is carried down to the subcutaneous tissues tangentially to the cyst wall and the granulation tissue surrounding the lateral tracts. Pilonidal sinus and tracts are thoroughly removed *en bloc* to the skin island, along with a minimal amount of healthy fat-bearing tissue, avoiding wide excision of the adjacent subcutaneous fat. Next, skin and subcutaneous fat from the right side are undercut and mobilized toward the left, across the midline, to cover the defect. The subcutaneous fat is undercut at the level of the deepest aspect of the sinus and at a plane above and parallel to the sacrococcygeal fascia. The width of the raised "tongue" of tissue is to the previously marked line of contact, in other words, the same as the depth of the cleft (Fig.9).

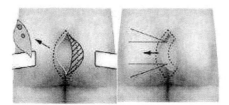

Figure 9- Bascom's cleft lip procedure

Adequate and careful hemostasis is subsequently obtained, and the wound is irrigated with saline and Povidone-iodine solution. If there is any skin overlap, some skin is removed from the left buttock to avoid any folding into the cleft. The inferior portion of the wound is rotated toward the anus to avoid a dog-eared appearance.

Application of inward pressure on the buttocks during closure is used to bring the edges of the wound together without difficulty. The wound dead spaces are tightly obliterated with interrupted 2-0 polyglactin sutures in one or two layers according to the thickness of the fatty tissue, without leaving a drain. The skin is closed with interrupted 2-0 polypropylene sutures with accurate apposition of the skin edges. Ultimately, the incision forms a line placed laterally over the left buttock, with both its extreme upper and lower edges on the left.

Patients can be discharged between the fourth and sixth postoperative days. Instructions for daily showers with P.ovidone-iodine scrub and at least bimonthly shaving (preferably with a depilatory agent) for a period of at least one year are given to all patients before discharge. Skin stitches can be removed between the tenth and twelfth postoperative days.

Bascom reported complete wound closure with the cleft lift procedure in 30 patients who previously had failures with other operations. There was only one recurrence at 2 years.

RHOMBOID EXCISION WITH LIMBERG/MODIFIED LIMBERG FLAP

A lateral advancement flap can be combined with a rhomboid type excision and rotational advancement flap. A rhomboid excision of the skin and soft tissues surrounding the sinus is made up to the level of the sacral periosteum. The gluteal fascia is then mobilized on its inferior edge laterally to allow a rotational tension-free flap to cover the rhomboid excision (Fig.10).

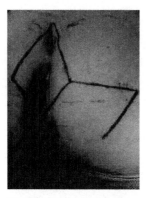

Figure 10- The rhomboid incision marking

The procedure- The sacral area is shaved, cleaned, and disinfected. Methylene blue is injected through the sinus tracts to mark all branches of the sinus. Then sinus tracts are resected *en block* with a rhomboid excision. The excision is carried down to the postsacral fascia. Then a Limberg flap is prepared from the right or left gluteal region. The flap includes the skin and the subcutaneous tissue. The flap is completely mobilized from the gluteus maximus muscle to prevent tension. After careful hemostasis with electrocautery, a suction drain is placed onto the presacral fascia, and subcutaneous tissue is approximated with 2/0 polyglycolic acid sutures. The skin is closed using interrupted mattress sutures with 2/0 polypropylene (Fig.11). Drains can be removed between 2nd and 5th postoperative day. Patient is usually discharged after removal of drain. The skin sutures are removed on 10th postoperative day.

Wound infection, seroma, wound separation, flap necrosis, and recurrence after long-term follow-up are the complications reported. The advantages of this approach are that the internatal cleft can be flattened and tissues can be approximated without tension. This technique also minimizes flap related complications such as ischemia and necrosis.

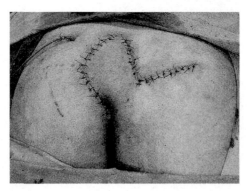

Figure 11- The limberg flap after closure

Dufourmentel suggested an improved approach to this rhomboid flap technique, where the apex of the main flap is situated more proximally than in the Limberg technique, and the angle of the triangular flap is less obtuse, thus allowing a less rigid transposing flap. The lower part of the suture line turns from the midline avoiding the need to lateralize the rhomboid incision as is necessary with the Limberg technique. The Dufourmentel flap can be reconstructed with lower tension because it requires less rotation of the flap. The narrower area between the defect and the flap does not cause any ischemia, because the subdermal plexus serves as the source of blood supply to the skin.

Several single-center studies have confirmed that rhomboid-shaped flaps such as the Limberg and Dufourmentel procedures have robust vascularity, with an absent or negligible flap necrosis rate, and that they are associated with the lowest morbidity and relapse rates. While Petersen and co-worker did not find any significantly different results among flap procedures in their pooled analyses, early wound failure and recurrence rates were systematically higher with V-Y advancement and Z-plasty than with rhomboid flaps.

V-Y ADVANCEMENT FLAP

V-Y advancement flaps involve excision of the sinus combined with a full-thickness flap in the shape of a 'V' with the ultimate post-repair suture line giving the appearance of a 'Y' after the flap is harvested and the defect is closed (Fig.12). The extents and directions of sinuses are determined in patients in prone position with the help of a lacrimal probe.

The procedure- Operative area is shaved with surgical clippers just before the operation and is marked in a rhomboid or elliptic fashion depending on the extensiveness of the disease followed by disinfecting with Povidone iodine. Using a scalpel, a full thickness of skin, including epidermis and dermis, is removed. Affected tissue, including all sinus tracts, are excised until fascia overlying the sacrum and lateral gluteal fascia and normal fat tissue are exposed. Electrocautery is used to avoid excessive blood loss during surgeries.

In V-Y flap technique, an incision is made as V pattern and the V-patterned skin is approached to cover the defected area as Y-shape. For this purpose, two equilateral triangles are drawn on two sides of the defect, and fasciocutaneous flap is prepared by going down to the gluteal fascia. Flap edges are cut in a bended way to be able to maintain a broader base. Mobility of the tension-free flap is ensured by incisions that are made in gluteal fascia and gluteus maximus fascias on the corners of flaps, when necessary. For the flap to fill the defect accurately, its base is undermined. The flap is fixed to the defect by appropriate movements. Primary closure is performed for the opening in Y's leg.

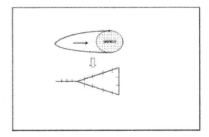

Figure 12- Marking for V-Y advancement flap

V-to-Y advancement flaps have been shown in several series to be reliable and effective in covering large pilonidal wounds. Schoeller and others demonstrated a mean hospitalization of 7.3 days and mean healing time of 15.3 days using this procedure. In their series of 24 patients, there were no recurrences with a mean follow-up of 4.5 years. To prevent recurrences in this series, the authors attempted to flatten the natal cleft by de-epithelizing the medial end of the flap and folding it under itself to fill in the wound defect (Fig.13). Recognizing the importance of closing the wound off midline, another study which performed V-Y advancement flaps in a group of patients, randomly allocated them into two groups: vertical suture line unrelated to midline and vertical suture line related to midline. Two recurrences in the group with the vertical suture line related to midline occurred at 15 and 22 months, whereas there were no recurrences when the suture line was placed off midline.

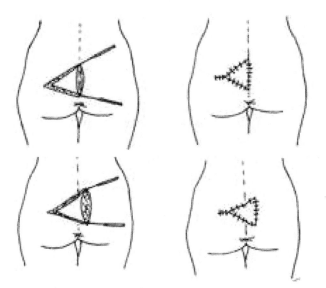

Figure 13- The advancement flap procedures in the midline and off the midline

Z-PLASTY

Z-plasty closure following excision of pilonidal sinuses was first described in the 1960s. Z-plasty has been adapted to the treatment of pilonidal disease and involves creating incisions in a 30-degree angle to the long axis of the wound to alter the depression of the natal cleft and allow primary closure. Subcutaneous flaps are then raised and transposed to close the excised defect (Fig.14). The procedure has been criticized, however, for a 20% incidence of tip necrosis. A series of 21 patients followed up for an average of 28 months showed considerable morbidity, including hypoesthesia in nearly every patient, and only 67% overall satisfaction. Patients frequently complained of discomfort, pruritus, and poor cosmesis.

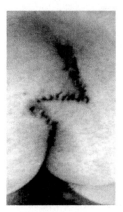

Figure 14- Z-plasty for pilonidal sinus

S-PLASTY

S-plasty has been favored by some researcher as they believe that it can reduce the tension on the excised wound, decrease buttock friction by flattening the natal cleft, and reduce the risk of fecal contamination by keeping the distal end of incision away from anus.

After shaving off the hair, S-plasty is designed, and the cheeks of buttocks taped apart. The longitudinal axis of incision depended on the axis of devitalized tissue or the secondary openings; the upper end of incision located on the same side of the secondary opening to reduce incision length. To improve wound healing by approximating fresh skin to the midline cleft, the lower end is incised away from the cleft. Excision includes the primary sinus and the secondary fistula opening or the previous incision and drainage site; completely removed unhealthy tissue without cutting into it. After achieving hemostasis, a suction drain is placed, and the tapes for traction removed. While the wound edges are being approximated with hands, lines are drawn perpendicular to the wound to match the margin (Fig.15).The wound is closed with mattress sutures of 2-0 Nylon through the epidermis, subcutaneous fat, and postsacral fascia. After subcutaneous tissue is sutured with 2-0 or 3-0 absorbable polyglycolic acid, the subcutaneous suture is knotted while the wound edges are being approximated with the neighboring nylon sutures, and then the nylon sutures are knotted from the upper to the lower. The patients are recommended neither lying supine nor sitting for 2 weeks to reduce the shearing force on sacrococcygeal area.

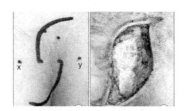

Figure 15- The S plasty procedure

GLUTEUS MAXIMUS MYOCUTANEOUS FLAP

Gluteus maximus myocutaneous flaps have been used in patients with extensive, recurrent, and complex disease. This procedure involves the mobilization of the gluteus maximus muscle to cover the excised defect. The assistance of an experienced plastic surgeon is often helpful. This is a large, well-vascularized flap that has the potential to fill large defects. Of concern is the potential for significant morbidity if wound complications occur. Additionally, this approach is associated with a significant hospital stay and limited short-term mobility.

The procedure- An oblique S-type incision is made. The extent and directions of sinuses are determined with the help of a lacrimal probe. All sinus tracts or diseased tissue containing tracts, including the subcutaneous, are excised up to the postsacral fascia. Both gluteus muscle fascia are incised vertically adjacent to the point where they adhere to the sacrum, and the fascia flaps are prepared approximately about a size of 3 to 3.5 cm. A careful hemorrhage control is performed by the use of electrocautery. Two separate sets of polyglactin sutures to pass through the gluteus muscle fascia of both sides and postsacral fascia are prepared. After loosening the adhesive tapes, the sutures are tied and are followed by separate subcutaneous and skin suturing. A light dressing is applied to the closed wound. Usually, no drain is required.

The procedure has been criticized for being too extensive because it sacrifices a deep functional muscle.

A single-sided innervated superior gluteal artery perforator flap has also been reported as a useful technique for covering large and recurrent pilonidal sinus defects following wide local excision.

PRE AND POSTOPERATIVE CARE OF THE PATIENTS WITH PILONIDAL SINUS DISEASE

The care of a patient with a post-operative pilonidal sinus should involve a holistic nursing assessment of the wound and the psychological effects on the patient which includes a discussion of various treatments and in the case of surgery proper explanation of the procedure as the patient might not be adequately prepared for the depth and size of the wound. Patients may also have fears about altered body image, self-esteem and anxiety in relation to pain. Recurrence and infection should also be discussed.

Pain assessment -Wound-related pain can be very distressing for patients and the strategies that can minimize this trauma have become increasingly recognized as an important element of patient care. The proposed strategies for assessing, documenting and managing pain in relation to wound care includes: preventive analgesia, explaining any procedures, positioning during surgery, avoiding exposure of the wound, time out, avoiding draughty, cold rooms, soaking the dressing before their removal and listening to the patient's views in relation to dressing changes.

Appropriate pain relief may range from regular paracetamol to opiates, depending on the severity of the pain, and should be provided on a regular basis to minimize discomfort, particularly post-operatively and at each dressing change. Consideration should be given to appropriate application and removal of dressings and analgesia should be offered before dressing changes.

Wound care- While surgically excised pilonidal sinuses are essentially clean wounds, the location can, however, predispose them to infection and thorough wound cleansing will be required at every dressing change. In the acute phase, warmed saline or even tap water can be used before the wound is redressed. For patients recovering from pilonidal sinus surgery, the key aims of wound management include: prevention of infection, reducing the risk of recurrence of the sinus, promoting healing from the base of the wound, swift re-epithelization with the best cosmetic result.

Therefore, selecting and utilizing the appropriate wound dressings is an important element of care. Initially, wounds which are being left to heal by secondary intention following incision and drainage should be packed with absorbent dressings, such as alginates or hydrofibres, which can be loosely inserted into a wound and are easily removed with warm saline or showering/bathing. These dressings are usually removed daily and can prevent leakage. Alginate dressings should be irrigated from the wound to ensure they are fully removed from the cavity and to avoid any residual fibers being left behind. They can last for 3–4 days but may also be changed daily.

Cavity dressings aim to keep the wound edges apart and prevent the development of superficial bridges and dead space in the depths of the wound. In order to reduce the risk of cross-infection, an occlusive secondary dressing should also be used where possible.

Dressing choices for pilonidal sinus include: Foam dressings, which take the shape of the wound itself. They can be applied over the cavity, maintaining a good seal and preventing leakage and infection. They can also be inserted into the wound cavity to offer absorption. Foam dressings allow the patient to manage their own wound care at home. They should be cleaned twice-daily to remove bacteria and a new dressing is needed every 1–2 weeks depending on the speed of healing.

Capillary action dressings can be applied into a cavity and the outer dressing changed regularly. The dressing lining the wound can stay in place for 2–3 days.

Anti-microbial dressings, such as honey, iodine or silver, may be used in those patients whose wounds are critically colonized or at significant risk of infection.

These should only be used for a limited time and a conscious decision needs to be made to continue with their treatment rather than just using them indiscriminately.

Topical negative pressure (TNP) therapy can be used for wounds with very high levels of exudates as management with dressings alone can be difficult. TNP works by removing exudates and bacteria from the wound via an electrical pump, which is attached to a suction tube fixated under a hermetically sealed dressing covering the wound.

Infection

Pilonidal sinus wounds are usually excised when they are infected and it is therefore possible that some organisms may still be present in the wound despite extensive surgery. Curettage offers the most effective method of removal of dead tissue, but as stated above, this can only be performed by an expert medical practitioner. Another possible cause of postoperative infection is the position of the wound and the presence of moisture and aerobic bacteria in the natal cleft area. The signs of possible infection include purulent discharge, excess exudates, friable granulation tissue, bridging of epithelial tissue across the wound, a malodorous wound, cellulitis, excessive pain and delayed healing. Implantation of a gentamicin-containing collagen sponge on the wound area in pilonidal sinus was found to decrease the rates of infection and recurrence while shortening the hospital stay.

It is important to remember, however, that some of these signs may be present in episodes of inflammation during the healing process and this must be taken into account when monitoring the wound for infection.

Scarring

Normal scarring should not be distinct from the surrounding skin and often occurs as a result of remodeling during wound healing. Scars continue to remodel for some time following wound closure and are not fully mature until about two years after the initial injury. Abnormal scars are formed due to a defect in the wound healing process and can have both psychological and physical repercussions. Appropriate wound management and good peri-wound care can assist in the prevention of scarring.

Health promotion

The patient should be encouraged to eat a well balanced healthy diet and drink 1.5 liters of fluid each day to try to prevent infection. Patients should be encouraged to reduce or stop smoking as this delays healing. Cleansing the wound and peri wound area should be encouraged and patients should be advised to take particular care with their personal hygiene as the area can very easily be contaminated with fecal matter.

Antibiotics

The routine use of preoperative antibiotics in a prophylactic role is unproven. Sondenaa et al evaluated the role of perioperative antibiotics using intravenous Cefoxitin versus no antibiotic in 153 patients undergoing excision with primary closure and found no significant differences in postoperative wound infections. Similarly, the efficacy of either oral or topical antibiotics in the postoperative period has not been clearly established in the absence of immunodeficiency, associated cellulitis, or concurrent systemic illness.

In summary, the routine use of perioperative antibiotics is unsupported. The use of antibiotics should be restricted to the presence of associated cellulitis.

AVOIDANCE OF RECURRENCE

The two main important treatment options to avoid pilonidal sinus recurrence include flattening of the anal cleft and keeping the area free of hairs. The idea of the flattening technique is to close the excisional defect of the anal cleft and to eliminate the cleft for which different surgical techniques have been discussed previously in this chapter.

Another important aspect is skin hair removal. Skin hair removal by shaving the natal cleft has been recommended for decades as an essential requirement for avoiding recurrence of pilonidal sinus. Various approaches have been adopted to get rid of these hairs including razor hair removal, waxing, use of epilation cream, photo-assisted epilation and laser epilation.

Regular razor shaving is supposed to be most commonly practiced method being cheap. However, certain issues are raised with this approach. Razor shaving procedure may cause microtrauma to the skin or enable skin hair to grow in the wrong direction. Most patients describe this as inconvenient and often difficult due to difficulty of access to the area.

Waxing techniques for hair removal carry a risk of severe burns and is reported to provide variable results. Hair removal cream does not provide reproducible results and can lead to allergic manifestations.

Another option is photo-assisted epilation. This treatment involves the administration of photodynamic agents, such as porphyrins or aminolevulinic acid, with subsequent exposure to light. However, available methods of photochemical destruction have achieved reliable hair removal only in experimental settings.

Lasers have been available for hair removal since 1996. Hair destruction by laser is achieved by selective absorption of light energy by the melanin in dark hairs. Short pulses of light treat a variable number of hairs within a target footprint. This is by no means a permanent method of hair removal despite media hype. Numerous studies have been carried out, and patients often report a 60-80% reduction in hair growth at 6 months. Multiple treatments are often needed and some believe only anagen hair responds. Multiple treatments seem to progressively increase the hair-free period in between treatments, and also decrease the percentage of hair re-growth. Hair removal is achieved in the most awkward crevices of the natal cleft using an easily directed light beam. The sinus is given an opportunity to heal by prolonging the hair-free interval. Complications are few, but a significant number of patients experienced discomfort with the procedures. Most required topical anesthesia. Rarely, blistering, hyper- or hypopigmentation occurs as a complication.

Laser therapy is by no means a cure for pilonidal disease. Removal of hair by this method can be an uncomfortable procedure and, although long lasting, is temporary. However, it represents an alternative method of hair removal, with a low complication rate.

POINTS TO PONDER

A number of different surgical approaches to SPD have been advocated. The surgical approach depends on the mode of presentation. For patients with an acute abscess, the sepsis should be simply drained with consideration given to a definitive procedure only where necessary. It appears that more than half of patients do not face any problem after abscess drainage and may not, therefore, require a definitive surgery.

Management of chronic pilonidal sinuses, however, is a far more controversial issue. The wide variety of surgical techniques described in the available literature reflects a lack of consensus as to an optimal surgical approach. Evidence supports both open and closed operative approaches with no major differences in complication rates. Open approaches with limited sinus excision are effective for patients with limited disease. If closed techniques are used, evidence supports placing the closure off the midline. Treatment must be adapted to the extent and severity of disease. Diligent, long-term postoperative follow-up and careful attention to wound care are essential.

Further reading and references

1.   Solla JA, Rothenberger DA. Chronic pilonidal disease. An assessment of 150 cases. Dis Colon Rectum 1990; 33: 758–761.

2.   Humphries AE, Duncan JE. Evaluation and management of pilonidal disease. Surg Clin North Am 2010; 90:113–124.

3.   Hull TL, Wu J. Pilonidal disease. Surg Clin North Am 2002; 82:1169–1185.

4.   Lee PJ, Raniga S, Biyani DK, Watson AJM, Faragher IG,Frizelle FA. Sacrococcygeal pilonidal disease. Colorectal Dis 2008; 10:639–650.

5.   Dogan y, Oguzhan S, Ahmet P, et al. Combined single step definitive treatment in acute pilonidal sinus abscess. Surg Sci. 2010; 1:24–26.

6.   Kepenekci I, Demirkan A, Celasin H, et al. unroofing and curettage for the treatment of acute and chronic pilonidal disease. World J Surg. 2010; 34:153–157.

7.   Thompson MR, Senapati A, Kitchen P. Simple day-case surgery for pilonidal sinus disease. Br J Surg. 2011; 98:198 –209.

8.   Lord PH, Millar DM. Pilonidal sinus: a simple treatment.Br J Surg 1965; 52:298–300.

9.   Millar DM, Lord PH. The treatment of acute postanal pilonidal abscess. Br J Surg 1967; 54:598–9.

10.   Bascom J: Pilonidal disease: long-term results of follicle removal. Dis Colon Rectum 1983; 26: 800-7.

11.   Gidwani AL, Murugan K, Nasir A, et al. Incise and lay open: an effective procedure for coccygeal pilonidal sinus disease. *Ir J Med Sci.* 2010; 179:207–210.

12.   McCallum I, King PM, Bruce J. Healing by primary versus secondary intention after surgical treatment for pilonidal sinus. Cochrane Database Syst Rev 2007;(4)CD006213

13.   Karakayali F, Karagulle E, Karabulut Z, Oksuz E, Moray G, Haberal M. Unroofing and marsupialization vs. rhomboid excision and Limberg flap in pilonidal disease: a prospective, randomized, clinical trial. Dis Colon Rectum 2009; 52:496–502.

14.   Gips M, Melki Y, Salem L, Weil R, Sulkes J. Minimal surgery for pilonidal disease using trephines: description of a new technique and long-term outcomes in 1,358 patients. Dis Colon Rectum 2008; 51:1656–1662.

15.   Bascom JU. Repeat pilonidal operations. Am J Surg 1987; 154:118–122.

16.   Senapati A, Cripps NP, Thompson MR. Bascom's operation in the day-surgical management of symptomatic pilonidal sinus. Br J Surg 2000; 87:1067–1070.

17.   Al-Khamis A, McCallum I, King PM, Bruce J. Healing by primary versus secondary intention after surgical treatment for pilonidal sinus. Cochrane Database Syst Rev 2010 ;(1) CD006213.

18.   Bascom J, Bascom T. Failed pilonidal surgery: new paradigm and new operation leading to cures. Arch Surg 2002; 137:1146–1150.

19.   Karydakis GE. New approach to the problem of pilonidal sinus. Lancet 1973; 2:1414–1415.

20.   Hosseini SV, Bananzadeh AM, Rivaz M, et al. The comparison between drainage, delayed excision and primary closure with excision and secondary healing in management of pilonidal abscess. *Int J Surg.* 2006; 4:228–231.

21.   Akinci OF, Kurt M, Terzi A, Atak I, Subasi IE, Akbilgic O. Natal cleft deeper in patients with pilonidal sinus: implications for choice of surgical procedure. Dis Colon Rectum 2009; 52:1000–1002.

22.   Bascom J, Bascom T. Utility of the cleft lift procedure in refractory pilonidal disease. Am J Surg 2007; 193:606–609.

23.   Mahdy T. Surgical treatment of the pilonidal disease: primary closure or flap reconstruction after excision. Dis Colon Rectum 2008; 51:1816–1822.

24.   Cihan A, Ucan BH, Comert M, Cesur A, Cakmak GK,Tascilar O. Superiority of asymmetric modified Limberg flap for surgical treatment of pilonidal disease. Dis Colon Rectum 2006; 49:244–249.

25.   Mentes O, Bagci M, Bilgin T, Ozgul O, Ozdemir M. Limberg flap procedure for pilonidal sinus disease: results of 353 patients. Langenbecks Arch Surg 2008; 393:185–189.

26.   Nursal TZ, Ezer A, Calikan K, To¨rer N, Belli S, Moray G.Prospective randomized controlled trial comparing V-Y advancement flap with primary suture methods in pilonidal disease. Am J Surg 2010; 199:170–177.

27.   Fazeli MS, Adel MG, Lebaschi AH. Comparison of outcomes in Z-plasty and delayed healing by secondary intention of the wound after excision of the sacral pilonidal sinus: results of a randomized, clinical trial. Dis Colon Rectum 2006; 49:1831–1836.

28.	Odili J, Gault D. Laser depilation of the natal cleft—an aid to healing the pilonidal sinus. Ann R Coll Surg Engl 2002; 84:29–32.

29.	Søndenaa K, Nesvik I, Gullaksen FP, et al. The role of cefoxitin prophylaxis in chronic pilonidal sinus treated with excision and primary suture. J Am Coll Surg 1995; 180:157–160.

30.	Aygen E, Arslan K, Dogru O, Basbug M, Camci C. Crystallized phenol in nonoperative treatment of previously operated, recurrent pilonidal disease. Dis Colon Rectum 2010; 53:932–935.

31.	Spyridakis M, Christodoulidis G, Chatzitheofilou C, Symeonidis D, Tepetes K. The role of the platelet-rich plasma in accelerating the wound-healing process and recovery in patients being operated for pilonidal sinus disease: preliminary results. World J Surg 2009; 33:1764–1769.

32.	McGuinness JG, Winter DC, O'Connell PR. Vacuum assisted closure of a complex pilonidal sinus. Dis Colon Rectum 2003; 46:274–276.

33.	Lynch JB, Laing AJ, Regan PJ. Vacuum-assisted closure therapy: a new treatment option for recurrent pilonidal sinus disease. Report of three cases. Dis Colon Rectum 2004; 47:929–932.

34.	Brook I. Microbiology of infected pilonidal sinuses. *J Clin Pathol.* 1989; 42:1140–1142.

35.	Harris CL, Laforet K, Sibbald RG, Bishop R. Twelve common mistakes in pilonidal sinus care. Adv Skin Wound Care. 2012; 25: 324-32.

36.	Jackie Stephen-Haynes. Pilonidal sinuses: Aetiology and nursing management. Wound Essentials. 2008; 3:128-33.

Chapter 6

OTHER PILONIDAL SINUS DISEASES

Pilonidal sinus usually develops in the sacrococcygeal area or other hair-bearing areas. It has also been described as an occupational hazard in barbers, especially when presented interdigitally. Occupational pilonidal sinuses tend to occur even in non-hair-bearing areas where there is no presence of individual's own hair. Pilonidal sinus occurs in many areas of the body such as web of fingers, penis shaft, axilla, intermammary area, groin, nose, neck following trauma during shaving, clitoris, sternum, suprapubic area, occiput, prepuce, chin, periungual region, breast, face or navel. Sporadic incidences of implantation of pilonidal sinus have been reported. The disease is mostly observed in hairdressers, but it has also been reported sporadically in other professions, as male sheep shearer, dog groomer, slaughter men or milker of cows. Short customers' hairs that penetrate the supple interdigital skin of the hands produce barber's disease. A synonym for pilonidal sinus is pilonidal granuloma. The histopathological appearance of the lesion is characteristic of a foreign body granuloma. An epithelial-lined sinus tract leads to an area of fibrosis and granulation tissue surrounding hair shafts.

INTERDIGITAL PILONIDAL SINUS

Pilonidal sinus of the interdigital spaces of the hand is a well-recognized occupational disease of male barbers .The higher incidence of the disease in male hairdressers has been attributed to those female hairdressers seems to be more diligent as concerns the cleansing of the interdigital spaces of the hands and feet. The interdigital spaces are susceptible to penetration by hair because the epidermis is very thin in this area; it is easily irritated by moisturizing agents and shampoos routinely used by hairdressers, while the tile-like formation of the cuticle can act as a barbed hook. Furthermore, clipped hairs are sharp as a needle, moist, electrostatic, adhesive, and preferably accumulate in the web spaces.

The exact reasons for the lesion are not known. However, several theories are offered. Hair penetration, negative pressure from finger abduction, recurrent infection and chronic infection are considered to be factors involved in the establishment of an interdigital web space sinus.

The lesion is produced by the penetration of foreign-born short hairs into the interdigital spaces of the hand. The hairs produce an inflammatory reaction and foreign body granuloma. They cause a sinus, and later a cyst. Through the sinus, the hairs get entrapped and may occasionally be expressed. Moreover, chronic, purulent drainage may occur. The structure of the lesions varies from epithelial-lined tract, cyst with surrounding foreign body reaction, to fibrotic cicatricial tissue. Most sinuses are asymptomatic and individuals may not even be aware of them. Although the clinical picture is usually benign, it can be complicated by repeated infection, which may require surgery. Abscess formation, cellulitis, lymphangitis and osteomyelitis are possible complications of barber's hair sinus.

Although thorough removal of imbedded hair might result in complete cure of the condition in certain cases, conservative measures in symptomatic sinuses have not actually proved to be totally effective. Dorsal metacarpal artery perforator flap is another choice with minimal donor site morbidity and which can provide robust skin coverage to avoid further penetration of hair in to web space.

Careful cleansing and drying of the interdigital spaces, as well as use of protective barrier creams, adhesive band-aid type strips, collodion, or fingerless gloves which maintain pulp sensitivity could prevent the formation of the disease. Moreover, hairdressers are advised to wear socks and shoes that do not expose the feet in order to prevent the formation of a pilonidal sinus on the feet. However, the main preventative method is the careful removal of any hairs that have penetrated the epidermis at the end of the working day.

UMBILICAL PILONIDAL SINUS (UPS)

Pilonidal sinus disease of the umbilicus is caused by hair penetrating the skin, causing a foreign-body reaction and development of a sinus lined by granulation tissue. Umbilicus could be an ideal area for PS formation since it is a depressed, moist and hairy area. Patients may not be symptomatic initially, but most complain of pain, discharge or bleeding at the umbilicus when symptoms do develop. With good lighting conditions and the help of an assistant to retract the skin of the umbilicus, hairs can be seen deep in the umbilicus and usually protrude from a small sinus. Additional diagnostic procedures are usually not necessary. Deep navel, an important anatomic variation, is common in such patients, which indicates a strong correlation with the disease. Additionally, inadequate personal hygiene is also noticed in the majority of patients. UPS occurs more frequently in young hairy males and hence is more common among students. The fact that young males prefer tight clothes may lead UPS to occur more commonly in this age group. Being hirsute is probably the most important predisposing factor. A strong family history of UPS was also noted. Wearing belt causes the hairs to be collected at the level of umbilicus and sets the ground for a moist environment, with the hairs piercing the skin. It is also thought that taking bath infrequently allows the hairs to be accumulated in umbilicus, inducing the development of UPS.

Simple extraction of hair from the sinus will relieve symptoms in most patients. Occasionally, incision and drainage of an abscess may be necessary. More aggressive surgical therapy should be used only after conservative management has failed. Surgical procedures in which umbilicus is completely removed, may cause cosmetic losses. Furthermore, losing the umbilicus may give rise to psychological misperceptions and make one feel as if he/she has lost connection with the mother, ancestors or even humanity. In order to avoid the psychological effects of such procedures, detection of etiological factors of UPS and determination of methods for preventing them would be more useful.

PILONIDAL SINUS OF THE PENIS

Pilonidal sinus of the penis is a rare entity, with very few reported cases. They clinically present as a classic case of inflammation with pain, local infection, and redness, but may also show chronic ulceration or a draining sinus or abscess formation. Pilonidal sinus of the penis is a rarely reported entity in uncircumcised men, the most common site being the region around the corona involving the foreskin for pilonidal sinus to occur in the penis, it is hypothesized that the coronal sulcus acts as a cleft where hair may accumulate from surrounding hairy areas of the patient or possible partner. The hairs are then driven into the shaft and prepuce by the mechanical forces and the rolling movement at the junction of glans penis and the uncircumcised prepuce. Simple excision with primary closure or healing by granulation tissue and sinus tract excision is usually the treatment for pilonidal sinus. If pus is available, it should be sent for culture and Gram stain. Long-term penicillin is prescribed after cultures and antibiotic susceptibilities to prevent sepsis. This is followed by circumcision to treat the underlying phimosis. In conclusion, pilonidal sinus should be considered an important differential diagnosis in a case of penile swelling, non-healing ulcer, or phimosis.

INTERMAMMARY PILONIDAL SINUS

Intermammary pilonidal sinus disease is commonly seen in fatty females with increased distribution of hairs. After the onset of puberty, sex hormones affect the pilosebaceous glands, and, subsequently, the hair follicle becomes distended with keratin. As a result, a folliculitis is created, which produces edema and follicle occlusion. The infected follicle extends and ruptures into the subcutaneous tissue, forming a pilonidal abscess. This results in a sinus tract that leads to a deep subcutaneous cavity. The direction of the sinus tract is cephalad in 90% of the cases, which coincides with the directional growth of the hair follicle. The laterally communicating sinus is created as the pilonidal abscess spontaneously drains to the skin surface. The original sinus tract becomes an epithelized tube. The laterally draining tract becomes a granulating sinus tract opening.

The sinus is caused by the friction of the skin leading to the embedding of the hair beneath the surface. The hair forms small cavities or pits, which are in truth, enlarged hair follicles, which go on to become sinuses. Bacteria and debris enter this sterile area, producing local inflammation and formation of pus-filled abscesses. In chronic condition, the sinus becomes an open cavity, constantly draining small amounts of fluid.

Although intermammary pilonidal disease may manifest as an abscess, pilonidal sinus, recurrent or chronic pilonidal sinus, pain and purulent discharge are the two most frequently described symptoms. In the early stages only a cellulitis or folliculitis is present. The abscess is formed when a folliculitis expands into the subcutaneous tissue or when a pre-existing foreign body granuloma becomes infected. The subcutaneous cavity and laterally oriented secondary sinus tract openings are lined with granulation tissue, whereas only the midline natal cleft pit sinus is lined by epithelium. The diagnosis of a pilonidal sinus can be made by identifying the epithelized follicle opening, which can be palpated as an area of deep induration beneath the skin.

Treatment for symptomatic sinus involves surgery to incise and drain the abscess. The surgery can be either wide excision and healing by secondary intention, excision and primary closure by sutures, or plastic surgery technique.

AXILLARY PILONIDAL SINUS

Sporadic reports of a pilonidal sinus in the axillary region have also been reported. This usually occurs in a hirsute person with the history and complaint of the intermittent small amount of leakage from axilla. Friction (abduction – adduction), suction, massage, shaving, pounding, minor infection and maceration are assorted mechanisms which play a part in causation of pilonidal sinus. On physical examination, a single or occasionally multiple sinuses which may or may not include any hair are noted. The sinus may or may not be expressing any discharge. The area around the sinus is edematous. Total excision with primary closure is reportedly an ideal treatment in this situation.

TUBERCULAR AFFLICTION IN THE PILONIDAL SINUS

Tuberculosis is a broad-spectrum disease that may involve pulmonary and extra pulmonary locations. Tuberculosis (TB) is a major public health problem, affecting 8 million persons per year worldwide. The global incidence rate of TB per capita is growing by ≈1.1% per year. Contrary to the increasing number of TB cases in developing countries, the number of cases in industrialized countries is stable or decreasing. Nevertheless, a decreasing trend of the total number of TB patients is seen with an increasing proportion of TB cases with extra pulmonary TB. Both the HIV epidemic and changes in population demographics, with rising numbers of immigrants, are being held responsible for this proportional increase of extra pulmonary TB. Extra pulmonary tuberculosis is responsible for 15%

of all cases of tuberculosis. In many countries; patients from Asian origin are known to have a higher incidence of extra pulmonary TB. Tuberculous infections have been increasing in incidence during the last decades for a variety of reasons, including increasing numbers of patients with immunity-depressive diseases, drug resistance, aging population, and health care worker exposure. As the rate of patients with extra pulmonary tuberculosis has increased globally in the last few years, the perianal localization is also increasing in similar proportion. Tuberculosis should be suspected in patients with complex or recurrent perianal septic lesions. The most frequently encountered perianal tuberculous lesions are suppurations and sinuses (Fig.1).

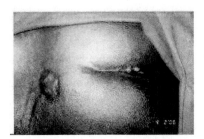

Figure 1- Tubercular pilonidal sinus

It is difficult to explain the possible cause of tubercular affection in the pilonidal sinuses. Cutaneous tubercular abscess can occur from extension of an embolism to subcutaneous tissue (such as pulmonary foci or direct skin inoculation) or from extension of an underlying lymphadenitis, synovitis, or osteomyelitis. TB has also been described following subcutaneous or intramuscular injection. Either the syringe, needle or fluid to be injected has been contaminated or the medical attendant has exhaled tubercle bacilli into the patient's skin, which are then introduced by the injection. It may be due to a direct inoculation from the stool of the patient, which may be containing tubercular bacilli. Another possibility is that the pre-existing sinuses get infected with tubercle bacilli either by way of finger or by the use of toilet paper. As tuberculosis in the pilonidal sinus is rarely diagnosed before operation on the basis of the clinical picture, the histological examination of the tract of the sinus is mandatory for the correct diagnosis. Novel diagnostic modalities such as adenosine deaminase levels and polymerase chain reaction can be useful in doubtful situations.

There should be a strong clinical suspicion of tuberculosis in endemic areas with such presentations as Mycobacterium is one of the causes of granulomatous diseases of the skin and subcutaneous tissues. Patients with such presentations are treated several times in the past by the family physicians considering it as boils or abscess. On occasions it is squeezed and drained and at other times it may be treated with antibiotics. The treatment often results in arresting the symptoms for the time being, but would recur after few weeks with similar symptoms and presentations.

Treatment of tubercular pilonidal sinus disease included two parts: conventional surgical treatment of sinuses and specific medical antituberculosis treatment.

Antituberculosis treatment is the mainstay in the management of tubercular sinuses. However, the ideal regimen and duration of treatment have not yet been resolved. Since 1982, the American Thoracic Society and the Centers for Disease Control have recommended a nine-month course of isoniazid and rifampicin for the routine treatment of TB in the United States. However elsewhere, a shorter course of four or six months of chemotherapy can be recommended for the treatment of perianal tuberculosis.

MALIGNANT CHANGES IN THE PILONIDAL SINUS

Common complications of pilonidal sinus include cellulitis, abscess formation, and recurrent sinus development. Less commonly, sacral osteomyelitis and meningitis can occur. Carcinoma arising from pilonidal disease is a rare complication occurring in the setting of long standing inflammation. Local recurrence is common and tends to occur early. Repeat surgery for recurrent disease may involve extensive resection.

Malignant degeneration occurs in approximately 0.1% of pilonidal sinuses. Males are most often affected, with a mean age at diagnosis of 50 years. The average duration of antecedent pilonidal disease is above 20 years. The mechanism by which malignant degeneration arises in a pilonidal sinus is believed to be the same as for other chronically inflamed wounds, such as scars, skin ulcers and fistulas. Immunosuppression and human papillomavirus infection may be predisposing factors to malignant degeneration of pilonidal cysts and may accelerate the transformation. Most of these malignancies are squamous cell carcinoma. Rarely Basal cell carcinoma arising in the pilonidal sinus has been reported.

Pilonidal carcinoma has a rather distinctive appearance, with the diagnosis frequently suspected by inspection, based on the presence of a long-standing and persistent pilonidal sinus with drainage, sudden rapid growth, overgrowth above the skin level, friability, ulceration, hemorrhage in the tissues, external bleeding, and most commonly, bleeding in sinus that has been present for many years (Fig.2).

Initial biopsy is to be performed to confirm the diagnosis. CT scanning may be useful in indicating the extent of the local disease and detecting any metastatic spread.

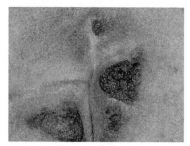

Figure 2- Malignant changes in pilonidal sinus

Treatment of choice remains en bloc resection, including the presacral fascia. Wide excision with tumor-free margins is performed with inclusion of skin, subcutaneous tissue, muscle, and, if indicated, portions of the sacrum and coccyx. Surgical treatment has reportedly yielded five year disease-free states in 55% percent of patients. Closure of the ensuing defect may be accomplished with mesh grafts, split-thickness skin grafts, or vascularized flaps, including gluteal rotation flaps and gluteal advancement flaps.

Some authors propose consideration of adjuvant chemotherapy and radiation to decrease the local recurrence rate. When radiotherapy is added to surgery alone, recurrence rates decrease from 44% to 30%. Re-excision of local recurrence resulted in some long-term survivals. Few successes have been achieved in patients who were treated with open and thick liquid nitrogen spray (cryosurgery) while monitoring the temperature through thermocouples.

POINTS TO PONDER

Pilonidal sinus disease is a common problem of sacrococcygeal region. However, it is also observed in other parts of the body. Though there are only a few reports about these peculiar sinuses in the available literature, they should be suspected in any chronically discharging, non healing sinus or wound. A clinical suspicion of malignant transformation or affection with tuberculosis in the endemic area should also be kept in mind to avoid any delay in the treatment and the final outcome of the disease.

Further reading and references

1. Ballas K, Psarras K, Rafailidis S, Konstantinidis H, Sakadamis A. Interdigital pilonidal sinus in a hairdresser. J Hand Surg [Br] 2006; 31:290–291.

2. Richardson HC: Intermammary pilonidal sinus. Br J Clin Pract.1994, 48:221-2.

3. McClenathan JM. Umbilical pilonidal sinus. Can J Surg.2000; 43:225–227.

4. O'Kane, H.F., Duggan, B., Mulholland, C., and Crosbie, J. Pilonidal sinus of the penis. The Scientific World Journal. 2004; 4 (S1):258–259.

5. Ferdinand, R.D., Scott, D.J., and Mclean, N.R. Pilonidal cyst of the breast. Br. J. Surg.1997; 84: 784.

6. Maor-Sagie E, Arbell D, Prus D, Israel E, Benshushan A. Pilonidal cyst involving the clitoris in an 8-year-old girl--a case report and literature review. J Pediatr Surg. 2010; 45:e27-9.

7. Sion-Vardy N, Osyntsov L, Cagnano E, Osyntsov A, Vardy D, Benharroch D. Unexpected location of pilonidal sinuses. Clin Exp Dermatol. 2009; 34:e599-601.

8. Uysal AC, Alagöz MS, Unlü RE, Sensöz O. Hair dresser's syndrome: a case report of an interdigital pilonidal sinus and review of the literature. Dermatol Surg. 2003; 29:288-90.

9. Pilipshen S J, Gray G. Goldsmith E, Dineen P. Carcinoma arising in pilonidal sinuses. Ann Surg 1981: 193: 506-12.

10. MircevaD, Miskovski A, Boskovski L, etal. Malignant changes in pilonidal sinus. Acta Chir Jugosl 1989; 36(Suppl): 778-9.

11.   de Bree E, Zoetmulder FA, Christodoulakis M, Aleman BM, TsiftsisDD. Treatment of malignancy arising in pilonidal disease. Ann Surg Oncol 2001; 8: 60-4.

12.   Gupta PJ. Pilonidal sinus disease and tuberculosis. Eur Rev Med Pharmacol Sci. 2012; 16: 19-24.

13.   De Martino C, Martino A, Cuccuru A, Pisapia A, Fatigati G. Squamous-cell carcinoma and pilonidal sinus disease. Case report and review of literature. Ann Ital Chir. 2011; 82:511-4.

ACKNOWLEDGEMENT

The author is indebted to all his colleagues, teachers, students and staff of his hospital who contributed in the form of references, drawing out figures, providing photographs of their cases used in this book. His thanks are also due to his patients who readily agreed to and provided him with their valuable post-operative feedback that proved helpful in his coming to certain conclusions described in this book.

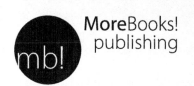
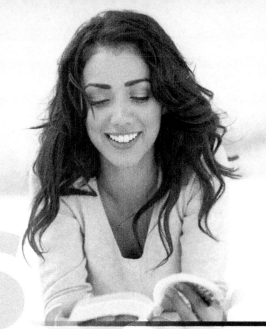

Printed in Great Britain
by Amazon